FIREFIGHTER FUNCTIONAL FITNESS

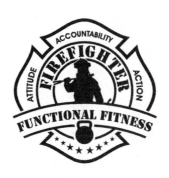

CW00952995

The Essential Guide For Optimal Firefighter Performance & Longevity

Dan Kerrigan   Jim Moss

Publisher: Firefighter Toolbox LLC
FirefighterToolbox.com
Book Website: FirefighterFunctionalFitness.com

Authors — Dan Kerrigan & Jim Moss
Introduction — David J. Soler
Foreword — Dr. Sara A. Jahnke, PhD
Edited by — Patrick Murphy
Technical Editors — Dr. Sara A. Jahnke, PhD, Dr. Karlie Moore, PhD

Library of Congress Cataloging-in-Publication Data available upon request.

Firefighter Functional Fitness / Dan Kerrigan, Jim Moss

Print-Paperback
ISBN-10: 0-9908442-4-2
ISBN-13: 978-0-9908442-4-2

eBook
ISBN-10: 0-9908442-5-0
ISBN-13: 978-0-9908442-5-9

Produced & Published By

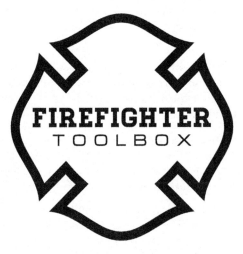

BUILDING BETTER
FIREFIGHTERS & LEADERS

Firefighter Toolbox is on a mission to build better firefighters and leaders by providing the mental tools needed for firefighters to reach their God-given abilities. The fire service is ever-evolving and we, as firefighters, are always facing new dangers within the profession.

DISCLAIMER

This book is designed to provide general information regarding the subject matter covered. The authors and publisher have taken reasonable precautions in the preparation of this book and believe the facts presented in this book are accurate as of the date it was written and published.

However, neither the authors nor the publisher assume any responsibility for any errors or omissions. The authors and publisher specifically disclaim any liability resulting from the use or application of the information contained in this book and the information is not intended to serve as legal or professional advice to individual situations or as a certification to anyone.

The recommendations, advice, descriptions, and methods in this book or program are presented solely for educational and informational purposes. Firefighting is a dangerous activity and occupation and could cause injury and death. This information is intended for certified firefighters or those looking to become a certified firefighter.

The authors, publisher, and Firefighter Toolbox LLC assume no liability whatsoever for any loss or damage that results from the use of any of the material in this book/program. Use of the material in this book is solely at the risk of the user, even if they are a certified firefighter.

Before beginning any exercise regimen, consult with a licensed physician to directly express any questions or concerns about participating in physical activity. If you are a firefighter, consult with a physician (preferably your fire department's physician) who is knowledgeable about the physically demanding tasks that firefighters perform. Only perform the exercises and movements found in this book if your fire department physician has approved you for full firefighting duties.

This book makes no specific claims about quantitative improvements in muscular strength, cardiovascular capacity, weight loss, flexibility, etc. It is not the goal of this text or the authors to diagnose, examine, or treat medical conditions of any kind.

For clarification or guidance on specific exercises and movements, consult with a certified personal trainer. As with any exercise regimen, the possibility of physical injury exists. If you engage in this program or any other exercise regimen, you do so voluntarily, understanding and agreeing to the risk of injury. In doing so, you agree to release and discharge the authors, the publisher, and Firefighter Toolbox LLC from liability.

TABLE OF CONTENTS

ACKNOWLEDGEMENTS

Dan Kerrigan

Tara, Sarah, and Ryleigh—For your unwavering patience, sacrifice, understanding, support, and love.

Mom and Dad—For your devotion, guidance, and the example you have set.

Jim Moss—For your passion in your efforts to reduce health-related line-of-duty deaths in the fire service, for your friendship, for your support, and for joining me on this journey.

Ken Battin—For your mentorship and support as a fire service brother and as a friend.

Rick Kline—For your mentorship, guidance, and ability to always set the right example. Every firefighter has a "first captain." That you were mine has had a positive impact on me throughout my entire fire service career.

David J. Soler and Firefighter Toolbox—For your friendship, support, and trust in me as a person and as a fire service brother.

The Firehouse Kitchen Table—For your unwavering support, encouragement, fellowship, and commitment to the constant improvement of our fire service.

The Brotherhood—For the support you all show as we fight for a healthier fire service together.

Jim Moss

God and Jesus—For their salvation, grace, and provision.

Ali—For your constant love, support, and patience.

Izzy & Maggie— For your love, inspiration, and joy.

Mom, Dad, and My Family—For always believing in me, supporting me, and pushing me to be the best I can be.

Dan Kerrigan—For partnering with me in the mission to make all firefighters more fit, healthy, and to combat the fire service line-of-duty death epidemic.

David J. Soler and Firefighter Toolbox—For investing and believing in me.

Metro West Fire Protection District—For being an organization where I can grow and thrive.

The Brotherhood & Firehouse Kitchen Table—For all of the support and fraternity from true brothers and sisters. *As iron sharpens iron, so one person sharpens another* (Proverbs 27:17).

ENDORSEMENTS

"Am I ready?" All firefighters are aware that they can be called to work at an intense and challenging fire at any moment, but *great* firefighters fully understand the difference between success and failure comes down to their everyday habits. They know their training, education, and fitness matter. We all have the time to improve our knowledge base as well as our ability to deal with the mental and physical stress of the job. Regrettably, far too many firefighters waste precious moments every day that they could instead use to prepare for *their* defining moment.

I promise you: At some point your body will be tested and your physical limitations will be exposed. It may be today, next week, or a year from now, but it's going to happen. Don't waste any more time. Ask yourself: "What can I do today to physically prepare for that moment?" If you struggle to find an answer, I'm confident that *Firefighter Functional Fitness* is the solution.

Frank Viscuso
Deputy Fire Chief
Kearny Fire Department, N.J.
Author, *Step Up and Lead* and *Step Up Your Teamwork*

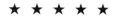

Firefighters must be jacks of all trades—especially with their fitness. We must have the endurance of marathon runners, the strength of powerlifters, the speed of sprinters, and the flexibility of yoga masters. It is very difficult to find a program that gives you the knowledge and tools needed to accomplish this—*until now*. With *Firefighter Functional Fitness*, Dan and Jim have nailed it! This book is a must-read for all firefighters!

Robert Owens
Lieutenant
Henrico County Division of Fire, Va.
AverageJakeFirefighter.com

Firefighter Functional Fitness is written to meet the needs of *any* firefighter. Dan and Jim address why optimal fitness is vital for all members of the fire service: volunteer, career, rookie, chief officer, retiree, man, and woman. Not only does it address why, the book also gives real-world solutions to address firefighter health and wellness. Dan and Jim give the information needed to address functional fitness for yourself, your crew, and your organization. I can think of no better fire service personnel to share knowledge for the betterment of health and wellness for our profession.

Susanna Schmitt-Williams
Fire Chief
Carrboro Fire Department, N.C.

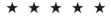

Dan and Jim have hit the nail on the head! They have given us the tools to successfully carry out our duty and to faithfully fulfill the oath we took when becoming firefighters. *Firefighter Functional Fitness* provides an outline for making the changes needed to reduce firefighter LODDs. This book educates the reader on the need for functional fitness and explains the crucial aspects that comprise it. Moreover, it provides the exercises, the nutritional foundation, the lifestyle choices, and many other factors that will assist any individual, organization, or department in developing and implementing a comprehensive health and fitness program.

Firefighter Functional Fitness will have a major impact on firefighter health, well-being, fitness, and injury prevention. I highly recommend this book to all our brothers and sisters in the fire service—from our newest recruits to our chief officers.

Collin Blasingame
Captain
Garland Fire Department, Texas
Cofounder, BlastMask
Coauthor, *The Station-Ready Rookie*
BlastMask.com

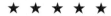

For firefighters and officers who are serious about firefighter health, safety, and reducing LODDs—*Firefighter Functional Fitness should be mandatory reading.* If you believe in reducing firefighter injuries and LODDs but need help addressing your fitness, this book will be your first step to getting started.

Firefighter Functional Fitness outlines very simple and specific methods to not only get healthy but also to be a functionally fit firefighter at a high level. This book is for all firefighters; because it's not about how much weight you can lift or how fast you can run, it's about how well you can perform the essential duties of firefighting.

Jason Hoevelmann
Battalion Chief
Florissant Valley Fire Protection District, Mo.
EngineHouseTraining.com

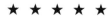

Firefighter Functional Fitness not only teaches firefighters why they need to be fit for the job and exactly how to do it but it also teaches them what not to do by dispelling some harmful myths that have been in the fire service and fitness industry for too long. As a scientist I'm excited to see a resource for firefighters that is research-based, and one that spells out a method that I know will be effective.

Dr. Karlie Moore, PhD
Exercise Physiologist and Nutritionist
Owner, Fit For Duty Consulting
FitForDutyConsulting.com

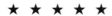

This is not your typical physical fitness book—*it is 100 percent geared towards the fire service*. Everyone from the rookie to the chief can benefit from *Firefighter Functional Fitness*. Any firefighter who puts these concepts into practice will be performing tasks on the fireground long after his or her colleagues have reached their physical limits.

Matt Valocchi
Assistant Fire Chief
Berwyn Fire Company, Pa.

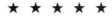

Functional fitness is much more than just being "in shape." Dan and Jim do an outstanding job not only explaining *Firefighter Functional Fitness* but also why it's critical, how to apply it to our job, and how to achieve it.

Through reading, understanding, and applying the lessons in this book, you will achieve firefighter functional fitness and have a long, healthy career that will last long after you stop crawling down hallways.

P.J. Norwood
Deputy Chief Training Officer
East Haven, Conn.

Whether you are a firefighter in the United States, Canada, or here in the United Kingdom, this book provides excellent information for firefighters of all ranks and ages. Dan and Jim are absolutely committed to reducing firefighter deaths through improved fitness, and *Firefighter Functional Fitness* is *the way* to help firefighters do just that.

Chris Blacksell
Deputy Chief Fire Officer
Humberside Fire and Rescue Service, U.K.

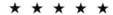

Firefighter Functional Fitness is for any firefighter, young or old, looking to increase their job performance and personal confidence! You don't have to be a fitness guru to implement the strategies offered. The functional fitness exercises outlined by Dan and Jim are designed specifically for the tasks firefighters carry out, which helps you to become an "occupational athlete" and be prepared for optimal firefighter performance!

Candice McDonald
Firefighter
Winona Fire Department, Ohio

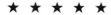

Firefighter Functional Fitness is the guide for proper preparation, fitness on the fireground, and for career longevity. We are industrial athletes, and it is imperative we prepare ourselves as such. This book provides a framework for fitness based around the duties that we perform day in and day out. The benefits reaped not only will make you better at your job but also have a healthier life.

Dan Shaw
Battalion Chief, Fairfax County Fire & Rescue Department, Va.

Doug Mitchell
Lieutenant, Fire Department of New York
Authors, *25 to Survive: Reducing Residential Injury and LODD*

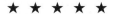

Firefighter Functional Fitness: The Essential Guide for Optimal Firefighter Performance & Longevity is right! Anyone who wants to be firefighter should be offered Dan and Jim's book when they receive their turnout gear. It covers everything a firefighter needs to know about functional fitness and how to put that knowledge into action. On behalf of The First Twenty and firefighters across America, thank you for your commitment to firefighter health!

David Wurtzel
Founder and Executive Director, The First Twenty
TheFirstTwenty.org

Firefighter Functional Fitness will benefit **all** firefighters who want to be more effective on the fireground. This book rightly acknowledges how fitness and health are interrelated. Functional fitness will improve fitness, enhance performance, and allow firefighters to be safer as they perform their work. **Every** firefighter who has sworn to protect his or her community and every leader who is responsible for the operational effectiveness of firefighters should read this book.

Dr. Denise Smith, PhD
Professor, Health and Exercise Sciences, Skidmore College
Research Collaborator, Illinois Fire Service Institute

Dan and Jim have done an incredible job of not only showing the importance of firefighter health but also providing a template that will empower firefighters to take steps in the right direction. Their commitment to your health radiates throughout this book. *Firefighter Functional Fitness* is a great place to learn the tools you need to prevent injury, increase performance, and build a healthier heart!

Jordan Ponder
Captain
Milwaukee Fire Department, Wisc.
Firefighter Dynamic Performance Training
FD-PT.com

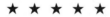

I gained invaluable information and workout ideas from reading *Firefighter Functional Fitness*. I incorporated numerous elements from the book into my workouts to ensure they are better focused on achieving and maintaining my functional fitness as a firefighter. My workout regimen is now more well-rounded than ever.

Firefighter Functional Fitness is an essential read for all firefighters looking to improve or build on their fitness for duty, as well as helping to improve their overall health.

Janey Reveley
Firefighter
Christchurch, New Zealand

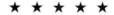

Firefighter Functional Fitness is amazing! This book is going to change the way the fire service views the importance of fitness! I'm excited for it to get in the hands of every firefighter across America.

As a career firefighter/paramedic and owner of BecomeFullTime. com, I am always giving aspiring firefighters tips on how they should train for the firefighter Physical Agility Test. This book is going to be my go-to reference for them! It will teach them the *why* and the *how* to get into top shape to become a firefighter candidate. This book is written for any firefighter at any level of fitness.

Brennan Palmer
Firefighter
Grapevine Fire Department, Texas
BecomeFullTime.com

Firefighter Functional Fitness is *truly* the essential guide to optimizing your performance and longevity as a firefighter. The benefits of your physical capabilities will extend far beyond the fireground in the form of decreased weight, increased energy, and an overall feeling of well-being. Execute what is in this book and reap its benefits for a long career and healthy life.

Robert Fling
Chief of Department
Dix Hills Fire Department, N.Y.
Founder and President, Facepiece On
FacepieceOn.com

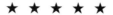

Dan and Jim do an excellent job of answering the *what, why, and how* of becoming a functionally fit firefighter, and they do so in a practical and unintimidating manner. From the rookie to the fire chief, *Firefighter Functional Fitness* is a must-read for any firefighter who wants to achieve optimal health and performance!

Mary Ellen Toscani
Firefighter
Berwyn Fire Company, Pa.

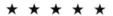

We, as firefighters, need to train our bodies for what we do. I am a believer that any exercise is better than no exercise. But why should we waste time on programs that are not designed to specifically improve firefighter performance and functional fitness?

Firefighter Functional Fitness is an *essential* tool for firefighters to improve their health, fitness, performance, and lives. Try it—see and feel the benefits!

Ken Battin
Director of Codes and Life Safety
East Whiteland Township, Pa.

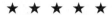

My biggest struggle prior to *Firefighter Functional Fitness* was lack of direction. I previously had many fitness goals in mind, but it was difficult to narrow down which I should concentrate on. *Firefighter Functional Fitness* provided a clear direction of where I needed to focus my fitness training and what would work best for me.

Krista Sayeau
Emergency Services Dispatcher
Ottawa, Canada

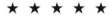

Firefighter Functional Fitness will help guide you on your journey to becoming functionally fit and maintaining your fitness. Wherever you are in your fitness journey, choose to make today the day you become a living example for others to follow as an advocate for Firefighter Functional Fitness.

Andy J. Starnes
Captain
Charlotte Fire Department, N.C.
BringingBackBrotherhood.org

INTRODUCTION

David J. Soler

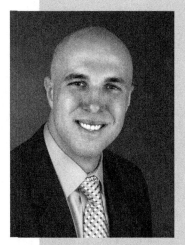

David Soler is the author of *Firefighter Preplan — The Ultimate Guidebook for Thriving as a Firefighter*, and the founder and publisher of Firefighter Toolbox. He is also the host of the iTunes top-rated firefighter training podcast called Firefighter Toolbox Podcast, where he shares powerful lessons from today's respected fire service leaders that will build and sharpen your skills as a firefighter and leader.

David is known for mentoring, training, and encouraging up-and-coming firefighters and officers. With more than 20 years in the fire service, he is a nationally certified Fire Instructor III, Fire Officer II, Rescue Technician, Haz Mat Technician, and his tenure includes serving in both career and volunteer organizations of varying size and complexity. Those who have read his books, listened to his podcasts, and implemented his strategies and principles have found themselves being more effective and successful firefighters, officers, and leaders.

THE PROBLEM: "AN UNFAIR HAND"

The deck of cards is stacked against firefighters and their health. When we took the firefighter oath, we never knew that our life expectancy would automatically be reduced by the hazards that confront us. Take your pick: *heart disease, obesity, diabetes, cancer, inhalation hazards, dehydration, overexertion, heat stress, sleep deprivation and disorders, traumatic and thermal injuries, psychological and emotional stress, PTSD, infectious disease, physical assault.* ... On and on, the list of hazards and "career side effects" continues with almost no end in sight.

When I signed up to be a firefighter, I knew it was an inherently dangerous job. However, I didn't realize that dying as a result of active firefighting (i.e. burns, structural collapse, running out of air, etc.) is such a small statistic compared to all of the other hazards and life-altering side effects of the job. I only know one firefighter who died from a "mayday" on the fireground on my watch. On the other hand, I personally know numerous firefighters and fire service mentors who have died from heart attacks and cancer before age 55. The statistics show that my experience is the accurate portrayal of what a firefighter will experience during a 20 to 30-year career.

I have interviewed many firefighters who have experienced the pain of losing fellow brother and sister firefighters. I find it imperative to bring this message to you with the *Federal siren roaring* and the *air horns blasting.*

MAYDAY! MAYDAY!

We have an emergency here! Realistically, you are more likely to experience pain and loss from the firefighter "career side effects" than you will from a fireground mayday incident. Now, we must still continue to diligently train on strategies, tactics, and firefighter safety to prevent a mayday from occurring at a fireground. We are doing well at keeping that number relatively low by improving fireground safety. Let's keep that up. However, the fire service as a whole (and at the individual level) must place greater emphasis on improving firefighter health and fitness if we are to mitigate the cardiovascular health epidemic.

CHANGES AND CHALLENGES WE FACE OFF OF THE FIREGROUND

Most of us don't realize there have been drastic changes to the foods we eat: *mass food production, genetically modified organisms, chemicals, stress, etc.* These changes adversely impact today's firefighters in a way that wasn't an issue 30 years ago. Studies and research have demonstrated the poultry and beef that we eat today is very different from that which previous generations of firefighters ate. In the standard American diet, we now have an overabundance of processed foods, fast foods, sugar, etc., that all cause negative health effects that didn't exist 100 years ago. These are just some of the examples of the many changes and challenges that we face off the fireground, as today's bravest.

THE SOLUTION

There are no two ways about it, we must make health, fitness, and nutrition fundamental parts of our "firefighter toolbox." To pave a road to career success, we must adopt health and fitness tools early on to develop the habits and disciplines of healthy firefighters. Let us live by these great fitness principles, and then pass it on to the future of the fire service. Let us lead by example in all things, especially by being healthy and fit firefighters. When it is finally time to hang up our helmets at the end of our careers, we will leave legacies worth following.

I know this is easier said than done. I know it's usually easier to grab a bag of potato chips, a donut, or a soda (which are chemically-altered to stimulate our brains and be addictive). We could continue to eat these unhealthy foods, but we're firefighters. We are made tough and can handle the tough things in life. We hold ourselves to a higher standard, and society honors us for that.

No more excuses. The standard has been raised. Now let us rise to meet the standard!

FIREFIGHTER FUNCTIONAL FITNESS IS BORN

Let me introduce Dan Kerrigan and Jim Moss—passionate advocates for firefighter health and fitness. As I have gotten to know them and how they live, I can say that they are realistic, and they are tough. They live the principles found in this book, and that is what I admire about them. Many times, Jim has gotten off a phone call with me to make sure he gets his "workout in." He has had personal tragedy and seen firsthand the results of a loved one dying too soon because of poor health and fitness habits. Being the student of great firefighters and success principles that I am, I personally wanted to learn from Jim on his motivation and discipline for his health and fitness. As I learned his methodology, I saw some great disciplines and truths that can positively impact the fire service. This is why I wanted him to produce a resource based on what works for him and for other firefighters to live healthy and fit lifestyles.

Then Jim tells me that I need to meet Dan Kerrigan. So, I meet Dan and instantly see his passion for firefighter health and fitness. As I have gotten to know Dan, I see his dedication to maintaining his health and fitness. At almost age 50, he has the body of a 20 year old. Dan and Jim partnered up to do some teaching on health and fitness that I had the chance to review. I knew they could bring a lot of value to the fire service in terms of their health and fitness knowledge, passion, and lifestyles. I knew that we, as up-and-coming firefighters, need better resources that are designed for firefighters on health and fitness. So it was a no-brainer to work with Dan and Jim to bring you *Firefighter Functional Fitness.*

THE METHODS AND METHODOLOGY

At Firefighter Toolbox, we provide you with the essentials of becoming a better firefighter and leader—*with no fluff.* We don't have time for the fluff. Dan Kerrigan and Jim Moss bring you the essentials of firefighter fitness with *Firefighter Functional Fitness!* With an easy-to-read format, it provides the knowledge and habits needed to optimally perform on the fireground, throughout our careers, and into retirement. It brings you their methods and methodology which are uniquely designed for the firefighting profession.

Firefighter Functional Fitness will address exactly what you need to get your fitness going (or continue the journey) in the right direction. Dan and Jim will keep you on the right path to reaching your God-given physical ability to perform on the fireground and beyond.

EVERY DAY IS TRAINING DAY

Remember: *Every day is training day*. Every day is an opportunity to build ourselves into better firefighters and leaders. Now, with *Firefighter Functional Fitness*, we can build ourselves into lean, healthy, firefighting machines. We need the mental tools, the physical tools (health and fitness), and the equipment to do this job. *Firefighter Functional Fitness* is the essential guide to physical success for the job.

Keep up the good work and make sure to leave the fire service better than you found it. May God bless you and protect you as you continue to serve others.

David J. Soler
Author of *Firefighter Preplan*
Publisher of Firefighter Toolbox

FOREWORD

Dr. Sara A. Jahnke

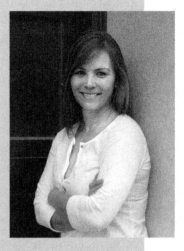

Sara A. Jahnke, Ph.D. is the director of the Center for Fire, Rescue, and EMS Health Research at the National Development and Research Institutes, Inc.

Dr. Jahnke has served as the principal investigator of two large-scale studies of the health and readiness of the U.S. fire service funded by the Department of Homeland Security. She currently serves as the principal investigator of a study on the health of women firefighters and as a co-investigator of several studies focused on fitness, nutrition, and health behaviors in both firefighter and military populations.

A passionate advocate and change agent, Dr. Jahnke works regularly with the International Association of Fire Chiefs, the National Fallen Firefighters Foundation, the International Association of Firefighters, the American Heart Association, and other national organizations to help improve firefighter health and fitness.

Firefighting is a team activity. While health choices are arguably personal for the average civilian, the fire service is different. As occupational athletes, the choices individual firefighters directly impact the risk other members of their crew face on the fireground. Choosing to be fit for duty is not just about personal performance. It is about your safety and the safety of your crew. It is about personal attitude, accountability, and definitive actions.

As a passionate advocate for firefighter health and wellness, much of my research is focused on identifying causal factors in firefighter sudden cardiac events and developing interventions to reduce their frequency. It is clear that research is increasingly identifying health risk factors as key predictors of injury and death on the fireground, making a focus on fitness and wellness central to a firefighter's job description. Obesity and low fitness have been found to be related to injury, cardiovascular events, and even non-cardiac fatalities incurred in the line of duty. I believe that taking a proactive approach to your own performance means not only training in fire behavior and fire tactics, but training the most important component of the fireground response—the firefighter. While improving fireground safety continues to be an ongoing and valiant cause, the focus cannot solely be at the operational level. As a firefighter, focusing on personal and crew fitness for duty simply must become part of the fire service culture if we are to decrease line-of-duty deaths and injuries.

This book brings together Dan and Jim's knowledge of health and fitness, experience on the job and their genuine passion for improving the health of their fire service family. A unique benefit that takes this resource to the next level is that it moves beyond the basic science and academic approach to fitness. By using their years of service and fireground experience as their foundation, they are able to distill the important details that firefighters need to know about functional fitness. Their experience in the varying levels of fitness of their fellow firefighters has resulted in a practical format that accounts for individual variation and needs, making fitness attainable for firefighters at any starting point. From the beginner to the trained occupational athlete, each section has useable Action Steps for every firefighter to begin making changes today, while also providing a roadmap for continued success. Firefighters who want to improve their health and fitness can easily assess where they are in the process, identify their first steps, lay out a plan for success, and get started.

While certain risks are inherent to the fireground and any emergency response, firefighters can and should take proactive actions to reduce their health risks considerably. *Firefighter Functional Fitness: The Essential Guide to Optimal Firefighter Performance and Longevity* is for any firefighter who cares about their own health, the health of their crew, and wants to improve their own fireground performance. It is essential reading for any firefighter that wants to decrease their risk of injury or death on the fireground and enjoy their retirement without disability. Lastly, it serves as the perfect resource to begin, revisit, build, expand, and grow as progress is made.

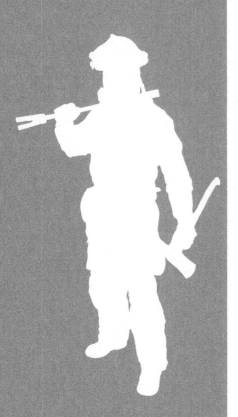

Being fit for duty is the most basic requirement for every firefighter— both career and volunteer.

—DAN KERRIGAN
AND JIM MOSS
"FOUR FUNDAMENTALS OF
FIREFIGHTER FUNCTIONAL
FITNESS"
(FIREENGINEERING.COM)

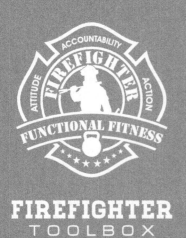

FIREFIGHTER
TOOLBOX

CHAPTER 1

FIREFIGHTER FUNCTIONAL FITNESS: A SIZE-UP

FITNESS AS A FIRE SERVICE REQUIREMENT

If there is one overarching theme to take away from this book, it is this: *Being physically fit for duty is one of the most vital and fundamental ingredients of being a successful firefighter.*

We are so passionate about this topic and believe in it so much that we are on a mission to assist all firefighters to become functionally fit and healthy so they can optimally perform on the fireground and in life.

For those of us who have gone through a fire academy or have participated in a new-hire testing process, one of the very first things that we did was complete a physical agility test. Before any skills training or classroom training, every aspiring firefighter typically has to pass a physical agility test to ensure that they have the *potential* to become a certified firefighter.

As David J. Soler has shared in *Firefighter Preplan*, in the heat of battle, fire does not distinguish between career, paid on-call, volunteer, male, female, young or old firefighters. Fire is a punishing and unforgiving adversary to *all* firefighters, regardless of their monetary compensation, gender, or age. Firefighting is physically and mentally demanding, requiring *all firefighters* to approach their fitness with the same level of commitment that they have for their fireground skills and knowledge.

As the old fire service adage goes, *you can never train too much for a job that can kill you.* We believe this truth is equally applicable to fitness training as it is to firefighter skills training and didactic knowledge.

Firefighting is strenuous, and if we want to do it safely and effectively, it demands an elite level of physical performance. It is a job that requires muscular strength and endurance, optimal cardiovascular capacity, flexibility, core strength, resiliency, and more. The fireground's physical requirements impact our bodies beyond physical strength in ways that we often do not consider—most notably when we exceed our cardiovascular limits. Additionally, we must also consider that we perform these tasks while being exposed to arduous thermal and environmental conditions.

Consider all of the different roles and actions firefighters perform on the fireground:

> Pulling and advancing hose lines
> Flowing water from hose lines
> Opening fire hydrants
> Wearing heavy and cumbersome personal protective equipment
> Forcible entry or egress
> Ventilating roofs, windows, doors, etc.
> Securing utilities
> Raising and climbing ladders
> Search operations
> Civilian rescue
> Firefighter rescue
> Roof operations
> Breaching walls
> Dragging, lifting, hoisting, and carrying heavy equipment
> Overhaul
> Crawling, pushing, and pulling

THE EFFECTS OF AGING ON PHYSICAL PERFORMANCE

Over the course of 20 to 30 years, a firefighter's time in the fire service can be unpredictable and grueling. Whether we are career, paid-on-call or volunteer, all of us want to maximize the longevity of our careers and retire "happy and healthy." Unfortunately, we constantly hear stories of retired firefighters who either die only a couple years after they retire or they are basically disabled during their retirement.

Due to the natural process of aging, our bodies undergo several physiological changes. Unfortunately, all of these changes work against our physical fitness as we get older:

> Muscle mass and strength decreases (3 to 5 percent per decade)
> Cardiovascular capacity decreases (10 to 12 percent per decade, starting at age 30)
> Flexibility decreases (increasing the risk and severity of injuries)
> Rate of metabolism decreases (accelerating weight gain)

Taking all of these factors into account, we cannot overemphasize the importance of every firefighter adopting a regular functional fitness regimen at the *beginning* of their careers. Doing so will have an enormous impact on an entire career *and* retirement. Even if you are a veteran firefighter who has neglected your fitness, don't worry—*there is no time like the present to start.* At any stage of your career, making small, positive changes in your fitness and nutrition habits will always reap benefits.

Firefighter Functional Fitness will make you more fit for the job, help keep your weight under control, reduce your risk of heart disease, diabetes, cancer, high blood pressure and high cholesterol, reduce stress, help you feel better, and add years to your life (while adding life to your years). By adopting *Firefighter Functional Fitness'* philosophy of balance and moderation now, you will reap big dividends for the rest of your career and retirement.

WHO SHOULD USE
FIREFIGHTER FUNCTIONAL FITNESS?

When it comes to fitness, firefighters will typically fall into one of five categories:

1. They lack the motivation to make fitness a priority.
2. They want to make their fitness a priority, but they lack the knowledge to start and maintain a program.
3. They have suffered an injury that physically hinders them from improving their fitness and maintaining a regimen.
4. They regularly exercise, but their workout program is not specifically tailored to the job of firefighting.
5. They are functionally fit firefighters who use *Firefighter Functional Fitness* to optimize their fireground performance.

Wherever you fall on this spectrum, *Firefighter Functional Fitness* will help coach you to either get out of the recliner and get started, stay with a program, or maximize your fitness by making it functional for the job.

Goals of *Firefighter Functional Fitness*

> Maximize firefighter performance through the improvement of cardiovascular capacity, functional strength training, flexibility, recovery, hydration, nutrition, and a lifestyle of moderation.

> Improve a firefighter's quality and longevity of their life, career, and retirement through functional fitness.

> Reduce the amount of firefighter line-of-duty deaths, job-related injuries, and health-related retirements.

> Reduce a firefighter's risk of developing cardiovascular disease, obesity, diabetes, hypertension, high cholesterol, cancer, and other related health ailments.

> Increase functional strength, capacity, endurance, and resiliency as they specifically relate to a firefighter's duties.

> Enhance physical performance and function.

> Achieve the best physical version of you.

Firefighter Functional Fitness is not a "traditional" workout program. Functionally fit firefighters are not concerned with having six-pack abs, a beach body physique, or aiming to hit a "perfect number" on the scale. Similarly, they avoid performing unsafe exercises and movements, lifting excessive amounts of weight, and trying to be stronger or faster than anyone else.

Like fire itself, *Firefighter Functional Fitness* does not discriminate. It is a program for every firefighter, whether career or volunteer. It works for all ages, genders, ranks, races, and backgrounds. We are glad you chose to take your health and fitness seriously, and we welcome you on this journey to optimizing your performance and longevity.

WHAT WILL HAPPEN IF I DON'T TAKE MY FITNESS SERIOUSLY?

Unfortunately, there are too many firefighters who take their physical fitness for granted. Conservative estimates state 70 percent of the American fire service is overweight. Obesity, diabetes, and cancer are all on the rise within our profession. If you have been in the fire service for any amount of time, you already know that more than 50 percent of yearly line-of-duty deaths (LODDs) are caused by cardiovascular events—primarily heart attacks. These statistics are just the tip of the iceberg for the health epidemic that the American fire service is currently facing. The more we continue to choose "recliner time" over "fitness time," the faster and deeper we will dig our own graves.

> **Even though firefighters only spend 1 percent of their time engaged in active firefighting duties, 32 percent of all firefighter line-of-duty deaths resulted during or shortly after this time."**
>
> —Dr. Stefanos Kales

Some may think firefighter fitness is a personal choice and its effects only have personal implications. The hard truth is our individual fitness levels affect our performance *and* our health. Our performance (or lack thereof) directly impacts fellow firefighters, the citizens we serve, and everyone's fireground safety. Our quality of health impacts our quality of life at home, it impacts our family, and it impacts the quality and longevity of our retirement.

33

So, if you're on the fence about making your fitness a priority, remember that it directly affects numerous important people besides just you.

   * To learn more on the health-related LODD epidemic, cardiovascular disease in the fire service and the cardiovascular strain of firefighting, please read Chapter 19 — *What Is Killing Firefighters: The Cardiovascular Epidemic.*

AFTER READING THIS BOOK, WHAT DO I NEED TO DO TO BE SUCCESSFUL WITH MY FUNCTIONAL FITNESS?

By reading this book, you have already taken a big step toward firefighter fitness success. You will now have all the facts needed to help you commit to firefighter functional fitness and make it an absolute requirement on a personal level.

Your personal *attitude, accountability*, and *commitment* to *act* are the three cornerstones for your success. We have written this book to provide you with the tools and concepts needed to take your fitness to the next level. We want you to accomplish this by applying what you read to your personal fitness program.

So, what's next?

Use this book to learn the fundamentals and also use it as a reference. Use it as motivation. Use it to teach your fellow firefighters why firefighter health and fitness are so important, and use it to become a champion for firefighter health and fitness.

Simply put: If you believe that being fit for duty and optimal physical performance are required of all firefighters and if you want to be a successful and effective firefighter, then *Firefighter Functional Fitness* is for you.

If you like what you read, we encourage you to check out FirefighterFunctionalFitness.com. Here you will find all the resources you need to continue on your path to optimal fireground performance through webinars, videos, training bulletins, demonstrations, explanations, and even live interaction with us. We look forward to working with you towards becoming a functionally fit firefighter!

THE AUTHORS' STORIES: OUR PERSONAL COMMITMENT TO *FIREFIGHTER FUNCTIONAL FITNESS* AND TO YOU

Dan Kerrigan:

I'll be honest. While I have always believed that fitness is essential to my effectiveness on the fireground and to my health in general, as a young man I had the same mentality that I see many younger firefighters display. When we are young, we believe we are *invincible*. Our focus is on becoming the best firefighter we can be, and this usually relates directly to our skills and knowledge.

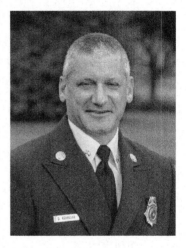

I never had a problem "keeping up" on the fireground when I was young. It was not until I got a little older that I started to realize a very sobering fact: *My 40-year-old body could not compete with my 20-year-old brain.* In this book, you will learn about the effects of aging that I began to experience firsthand. Several years ago, there was an arson crisis in my area. We were seeing a lot of work. A lot. It was tragic from a community standpoint, but it was also a personal eye-opener for me. I noticed that I was not able to recover as quickly as I used to, both on the fireground and in between fires. I was tired. I was sore. I found myself more reliant on that adrenaline boost than ever before.

Fortunately for me, I discovered Russian kettlebells. I immediately realized how "functional" the movements were and how effective the training was. I am not here to "sell" kettlebells, but I am here to tell you that this was *my* "ah-ha" moment. I have since conducted applied research and have piloted functional fitness studies. I have implemented a functional fitness program at my department. I use The Big 8 of *Firefighter Functional Fitness* every day as the backbone of my fitness training. I have also learned to be more sensible about what I eat and focus on proper hydration and rest.

As a firefighter, I have always been very aggressive. I have always enjoyed the physical aspects of the work. As a chief officer, I have also come to recognize how much my own physical fitness has a direct bearing on how I handle stress and my ability to think and act decisively under pressure. Now, at nearly 50 years old, I can say without fear of contradiction that I am in the best *functional* shape of my career and my life. The proof is in performance. I see and feel it personally, and I can also see it in the firefighters in my department. They take functional fitness seriously, and they routinely outwork and outperform anyone on the fireground who does not take the same approach.

Firefighter Functional Fitness works. It is a comprehensive approach that you can use to improve and maintain your fitness for duty. By adopting the principles found in this book, you will be demonstrating to your fellow firefighters, community, and, most importantly, your family that you are serious about taking care of yourself.

Jim Moss:

Fitness has always been an important part of my life—even since childhood. I started to get serious about my fitness while I was in college; however, I narrowly focused my fitness on just improving my physique. Like almost everyone else, I was originally taught a strength and conditioning model that emphasized strength training based on body parts and muscles groups (i.e. bench press for "chest," leg extensions for "quads," etc.). Unfortunately, that fitness regimen did not fully prepare me for real-life function and performance.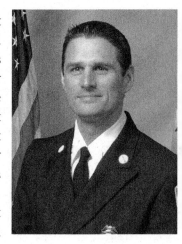

On the path towards preparing for the fire academy, I started to gear my fitness specifically for *firefighter performance*. I would wear a backpack with 50 pounds of weight and do high-intensity interval training on a stair climber. I also used the cable resistance machines to simulate pulling a hose line and hoisting tools. I used pushing, pulling, carrying, lifting, and dragging exercises to maximize my functionality as a firefighter.

During a year-long period on the job, I unfortunately decided to strictly focus on strength training in an effort to *"bulk up."* Regrettably, I was neglecting my cardiovascular capacity, flexibility, core strength, and not incorporating enough rest into my weekly workouts. What resulted was a strained chest muscle and an injured shoulder. After those healed, I made it a goal to make my fitness specifically *functional* for the job of firefighting. I incorporated all aspects of The Big 8, while balancing rest, recovery, better hydration and improved nutrition.

At age 35, I can honestly say I am in the best shape of my life. With concepts found in *Firefighter Functional Fitness*, I have found balance and moderation in my fitness and health. I will admit I am not the biggest or strongest firefighter; however, I have recorded the fastest time on my fire department's physical agility assessment for the past couple of years. As it pertains to the fireground, I have optimized my performance and I seldom need to rest. After a fire, I notice that my body and energy recover quickly and I am immediately ready for the next fire.

TRAIN LIKE YOU FIGHT; FIGHT LIKE YOU TRAIN

We firmly believe the greater we can make our fitness training mimic the intensity and realism of fireground activities, and the more emphasis we place on lifestyle choices that reflect a moderate, sensible, healthy approach, the less margin for failure we expose ourselves to when performing on the fireground.

We must not simply survive the fireground, we must be able to thrive on the fireground. It all starts with a foundation of functional fitness.

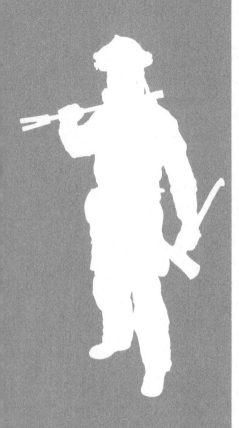

Are you a firefighter?

Do you want to be a firefighter?

Then train like a firefighter is supposed to train.

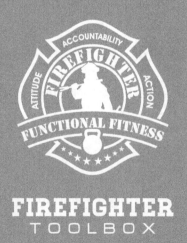

FIREFIGHTER
TOOLBOX

CHAPTER 2

FIREFIGHTER FUNCTIONAL FITNESS DEFINED

Firefighter Functional Fitness is a practical and comprehensive approach to firefighter fitness that uses real-life activities, positions, and exercises to best prepare us for optimal firefighter performance. In addition to physical exercise, it also incorporates recovery, hydration, nutrition and a lifestyle of moderation to develop a holistic approach to fitness, which not only improves fireground performance but also better health overall.

Most definitions of the word "fitness" will use general terms like *health*, *conditioning*, *exercise*, and *strength*. These terms can be ambiguous, and they leave a lot of room for individual interpretation. Unfortunately, they tend to make people only think of specific (yet limited) components of overall health and fitness.

The concept of personal fitness is subjective, and its meaning may vary from person to person. For example, a marathoner's idea of fitness may translate to running 20 miles at a 6-minute pace. On the other hand, a bodybuilder may rate their fitness based on how much muscle they have gained or by their physique. On the other end of the spectrum, an individual with chronic heart disease may see fitness as their ability to perform daily activities without becoming short of breath (e.g. taking out the trash, walking up a flight of stairs, etc.). Clearly, the idea of "fitness" is relative, and it is based on an individual's goals and ideologies.

As numerous firefighter fitness advocates have preached before, firefighters are *occupational athletes*. Using this as our model, let's examine how other serious athletes train. Consider gymnasts, football players, and the like. *These athletes tailor their physical fitness regimens for very specific performance requirements.* For example, gymnasts perform flexibility training, as well as ring, beam, and vault exercises. As for football players, they do sprints, explosive strength training, and applicable field exercises.

We firmly believe that as firefighters, we must specifically tailor our fitness training to best prepare us for firefighting duties. What sense does it make for a firefighter to only do strength exercises or to *only* do cardiorespiratory training? Just as much sense as it would make for a firefighter to train like a gymnast or football player.

When all is said and done, firefighters have very specific job functions that require specific functional training.

THE 4 PILLARS OF FIREFIGHTER FUNCTIONAL FITNESS

There are four pillars of *Firefighter Functional Fitness* that form the *strategies* of optimizing fireground performance. When applied appropriately and consistently, they give firefighters the greatest opportunity for health and fitness success.

1. Physical fitness
2. Recovery and rest
3. Hydration
4. Nutrition and lifestyle

Within each of these pillars, we will introduce specific concepts. These functional fitness *tactics* will teach you, guide you, and help you to develop yourself into a firefighter of elite performance. As we have said before, focusing on limited aspects of firefighter fitness will only provide limited results. It is important to understand that the best way to achieve the best version of you is to adopt and apply the tactics found in each of these pillars.

PILLAR 1: PHYSICAL FITNESS

Physical fitness is the most thought about pillar by firefighters who try to take their performance seriously. In simplistic terms, physical fitness involves improving or increasing physical strength, muscular endurance, flexibility, and cardiovascular capacity as a means to improve health and functionality.

There are many paths to accomplish these tasks. However, in order to accomplish firefighter fitness objectives in the most efficient manner, we have developed **The Big 8** of *Firefighter Functional Fitness*. The Big 8 will help you improve your fitness for duty in a simple and systematic manner. It brings together eight functional categories that are directly applicable to firefighters. In this book, we will break down each category and provide specific exercises and movements to improve your fireground performance.

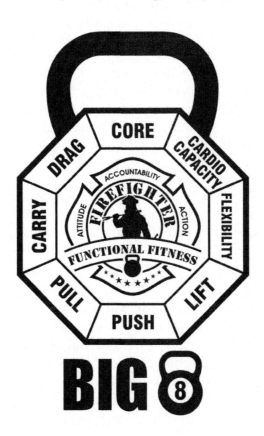

PILLAR 2: RECOVERY AND REST

If we do not allow our bodies the time they need to recharge and recover from strenuous activity, we run a greater risk (especially over time) of suffering detrimental physical and mental effects. Passive and active recovery are two primary methods we will use to help us maximize the results from our workouts.

Rest and sleep are two of the most important aspects of passive recovery. Instead of working out every day of the week, we must incorporate adequate rest to balance the equation. This includes resting in between workout sessions to rebuild and repair our muscles. Depending on our current conditioning level (i.e. how well we are "in-shape"), we will have to find the right balance between "workout days" and "rest days." For example, a deconditioned firefighter may only be able to exercise two to three days per week initially. On the other hand, the well-conditioned, "functionally fit" firefighter can realistically work out five to six days per week.

To maximize our functional fitness, we must incorporate adequate sleep. Now, it may seem like the words "firefighter" and "sleep" together are an oxymoron, but firefighters must place greater emphasis on getting a good night's sleep. Adequate sleep has been proven to decrease the risk of developing heart disease, diabetes, kidney disease, and obesity. Additionally, quality sleep aids in muscle repair and building muscular strength.

Active recovery methods include a post-workout cool-down, self-myofascial release (foam rolling), various forms of stretching, massage, and optimal hydration and nutrition. Cool-downs are used to gradually get our bodies to return back to a normal resting state after a strenuous workout. They should last 5 to 10 minutes and blend light cardiorespiratory activity (e.g. walking), foam rolling, and static stretching. When used in warm-ups, cool-downs, and as needed in between workouts, foam rolling breaks up muscle adhesions, decreases muscle soreness, and wards off fatigue and injury. Lastly, we should consider a weekly (or biweekly) massage to relieve physical and mental stress. We will provide specific methods to improve your quality of rest and your recovery from exercise and from other strenuous activities such as firefighting.

PILLAR 3: HYDRATION

Hydration methods are the ways we maintain and restore appropriate fluid balance in our bodies. The effort we put into taking care of our bodies and how well we keep our vital systems functioning cannot be overstated. At an incident, firefighters can lose almost 2 liters per hour while participating in active firefighting duties. Unfortunately, most firefighters do not properly hydrate throughout the day, nor do they fully rehydrate after an incident. This lack of hydration impacts organ and body system health as well as physical performance.

What many firefighters do not know is that dehydration increases the risk of heart attacks, strokes, cancer, and other health conditions. When we are dehydrated, we cannot sufficiently maintain a safe core temperature, our blood volume decreases, and our blood becomes too thick. All of these factors contribute to the formation of blood clots and blockages within our cardiovascular system.

Unfortunately, many firefighters do not fully grasp the importance of proper hydration until they are already suffering the signs and symptoms of dehydration. Firefighting is a profession that requires firefighters to be proactive in every area—training, pre-planning, maps, etc. As it pertains to fitness and physical performance, we must also take a proactive approach to our hydration. This means drinking enough quality fluids throughout the day to maintain *euhydration*—the state of normal body water content. This does not mean we are limited to *only* drinking water as our primary source of fluids. We can also obtain sufficient fluids from quality fruits, vegetables, and other foods.

The prevalence of cancer in the fire service is at an all-time high. Even if we wear the appropriate respiratory protection at a fire, we still absorb smoke's carcinogens through our skin, into our bloodstream, and into our vital organs. Euhydration and post-incident rehydration help prevent cancer by increasing cellular oxygenation, boosting immune system function, reducing the risk of diabetes and obesity (risk factors for cancer), and by flushing toxins out of our bodies. Later in this book, we will dedicate a chapter to teaching you how to be proactive about your hydration and give you tips to maintain proper body fluid balance.

PILLAR 4: NUTRITION AND LIFESTYLE

As previously discussed, obesity, diabetes, and cardiovascular disease are all on the rise in the American fire service. Sedentary behavior has a role in this epidemic, but the primary culprit is a firefighter's unhealthy dietary choices. If we are going reduce the number of firefighter cardiac events and line-of-duty deaths, it has to start in the kitchen.

> **"If we are going reduce the number of firefighter cardiac events and line-of-duty deaths, it has to start in the kitchen."**

No matter how much effort we put into improving our physical conditioning, what (and how much) we choose to eat and drink will likely end up having the greatest impact on our performance and long-term health. Much like putting premium fuel into a luxury sports car, we must feed our bodies premium "fuels" to maximize their output and longevity.

To be functionally fit, our bodies need the right blend of healthy macronutrients: Fats, carbohydrates, proteins, and fiber. These are not only critical building blocks to optimizing our fireground performance, but they are also essential elements to improving our general health, the way we feel, and the longevity and quality of our careers and subsequent retirements.

Many people find the topic of nutrition to be confusing and imposing. We are not nutritionists, but we will give you a common-sense approach that stresses moderation and balance. We will tell you which foods are best, which foods to consume minimally, and we will give you practical tips and guidelines to make smart choices.

On the fireground, sound strategies and tactics combine to help firefighters meet their objectives and achieve high levels of success. Consider The 4 Pillars of *Firefighter Functional Fitness* your strategies for fitness success, and use the tactics found within each or them to help you to reach your own success in fitness and health.

ACTION STEPS:

1. **Know that The 4 Pillars of *Firefighter Functional Fitness* are:**

   › **Physical fitness**

   › **Recovery and rest**

   › **Hydration**

   › **Nutrition and lifestyle**

2. **Keep reading *Firefighter Functional Fitness* to learn how to adopt and implement The 4 Pillars into your workout routine and daily life.**

3. **Make one small improvement in your diet or hydration today to increase your functional fitness.**

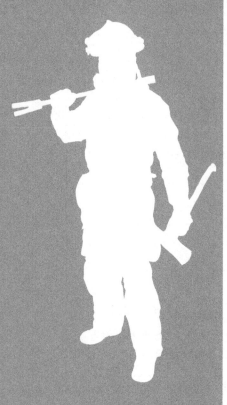

Even in small doses, regular physical activity can help prevent, treat, and in some cases even cure more than 40 of the most common chronic health conditions encountered, as well as reduce healthcare costs and improve the quality and quantity of life.

—NATIONAL ACADEMY OF SPORTS MEDICINE

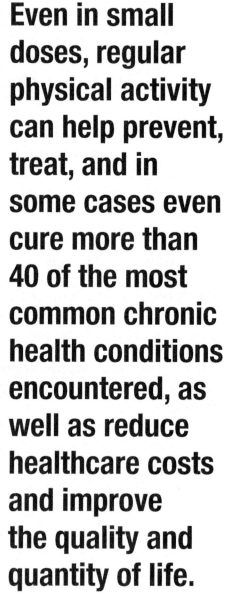

ACCOUNTABILITY
FIREFIGHTER
ATTITUDE
ACTION
FUNCTIONAL FITNESS

FIREFIGHTER
TOOLBOX

CHAPTER 3
PILLAR 1: PHYSICAL FITNESS

The first pillar of *Firefighter Functional Fitness* is **physical fitness**. Our physical fitness efforts will always focus on optimizing our:

> ‣ Core strength
> ‣ Cardiovascular capacity
> ‣ Flexibility
> ‣ Muscular strength, endurance, and power

We will invest the majority of our efforts discussing physical fitness, because it plays the principal role in achieving our functional fitness and performance as firefighters.

For the longest time, firefighters who worked out primarily focused on strength training (i.e. lifting weights)—placing little to no focus on core strength, aerobic capacity or flexibility. Compounding the problem, firefighters were originally taught a strength and conditioning model that focused on specific muscles of the body—*chest, shoulders, triceps, biceps, abs, etc*. This "bodybuilding mentality" encouraged firefighters to focus more on their physique and strength instead of real-life function and performance.

Now, if you are a firefighter whose primary fitness goals are to "gain mass" and "get ripped," we want to re-emphasize *Firefighter Functional Fitness* is probably not for you. However, if you are a firefighter who wants to improve all aspects of your *performance*, then please join us on this journey to make your fitness *functional*.

Firefighter Functional Fitness focuses on building firefighters into optimal fireground performers. Pillar 1 is more than just strength training. All four components in this first pillar combine to optimize our health, fitness, and performance.

Consider The Big 8 your definitive set of physical fitness tactics to help accomplish your functional fitness strategy. Using The Big 8 concept as our model, we emphasize a comprehensive and balanced approach to firefighter fitness.

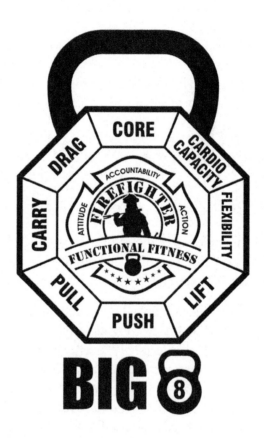

Core, cardiovascular capacity, and flexibility are the first three components of The Big 8. We purposely chose to discuss these three categories first because the majority of firefighters' fitness routines are severely lacking in these areas. Don't make the same mistake as others. Implement core, cardiovascular capacity, and flexibility into your program—*we cannot emphasize this enough*.

The remainder of The Big 8 incorporates strength training by emphasizing functional *movements*. These performance-based movements are functional because they directly relate to important and practical fireground tasks. Instead of using the archaic and impractical strength and conditioning model that focused on specific muscle groups, we want all firefighters to rethink how they approach functional strength. As functionally fit firefighters, we must be well-rounded and physically prepared for the fireground.

Throughout this book, we will examine each element of The Big 8, explain how they relate to our functional fitness, and provide guidance on how to incorporate them into fitness routines.

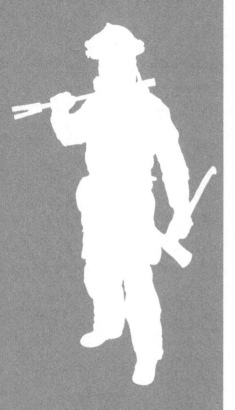

Our core is our center, and it is essentially the foundation of our functional fitness.

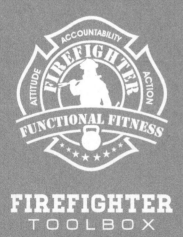

FIREFIGHTER
TOOLBOX

CHAPTER 4

THE BIG 8: CORE STRENGTH

WHAT IS CORE STRENGTH?

The core consists of the muscles in the front, back, and sides of the torso. There are approximately 20 muscles that work together to help the torso flex, extend, twist, and bend. In the realm of fitness, some may think core strength simply translates to strong abdominal muscles or a nice set of "six-pack abs." However, core strength is what provides integrity, stability, and proper posture to the spine.

WHY IS CORE STRENGTH IMPORTANT FOR FIREFIGHTERS?

When it comes to functional fitness, most firefighters tend to overlook core strength. As mentioned, most firefighters (who exercise regularly) usually focus on strength training of all body areas except for the core (i.e. chest, biceps, triceps, shoulders, legs, etc.). Unfortunately, any fitness regimen that neglects core strength is missing a big piece of the puzzle.

> **Any fitness regimen that neglects core strength is missing a big piece of the puzzle."**

In the course of firefighting duties, we quickly twist, bend, and contort our bodies in awkward positions. Furthermore, we perform these movements with an excessive amount of weight and with PPE ensembles that restrict our range of motion.

Our core is our center, and it is essentially the foundation of our functional fitness as firefighters. A weak, inflexible, and unbalanced core will adversely affect our upper and lower-body strength, agility, and performance. Like links of a chain, our core connects our legs to our upper body and arms. If our core is weak and nonproductive, the other parts of our body will be compromised. Core strength is also necessary for optimal balance, stability, flexibility, posture, and body ergonomics. All of these elements combine to help us function at optimal capacity.

Finally, let's not forget: The primary injuries for firefighters are strains and sprains. Lifting, pulling, pushing, dragging, and carrying heavy objects will take their toll on our backs and bodies if we do not properly strengthen all of our core. Every firefighter wants to have a healthy career and retirement—a strong core goes a long way to reducing the incidence and severity of injuries during a firefighter's career.

HOW TO BUILD CORE STRENGTH

Part 1: 4 Rules for Safe and Effective Core Strength Training

Rule 1: Engage the Core

Before we present specific core-strengthening exercises, we must explain what it means to "engage the core." Many of us have heard this phrase before but may not know what it means or how to do it. *Engaging the core* simply translates to tightening our core muscles to increase stability in the torso. We do this by physically contracting our core muscles and mentally focusing on these muscles during an exercise.

To accomplish this, imagine someone is about to punch your stomach. To brace for the impact of the punch, you would contract your core muscles to protect the abdomen. During our core exercises, we don't need to engage the core at 100 percent effort. Rather, we should engage it just enough to stabilize the torso.

Engaging our core is the foundation of many other functional movements—lifting, dragging, pushing, pulling, and carrying. Doing so encourages proper form, body mechanics, and helps reduce the risk of a back injury when executing these movements.

Rule 2: Go Slow — *Slow Is Smooth, Smooth Is Strong*

Building core strength is not about speed or how fast we can finish an exercise. When first starting to build core strength, perform exercises in a slow and controlled manner. Beginners should focus on core exercises that build stability and balance. These include isometric exercises. An isometric exercise is a strength training exercise in which the length of a muscle and a joint's angle do not change. Examples of isometric core exercises include planks, side planks, bridge pose, etc. Once you are able to perform three rounds of these exercises (for 30 seconds or more and with good form), you can venture into other core exercises that require dynamic movement.

Rule 3: Avoid Hyperextension and Hyperflexion of the Spine

According to Dr. Karlie Moore of *Fit For Duty Consulting*, firefighters should avoid hyperextension and hyperflexion of the spine. Hyperextension means that the spine is bending too far backward—examples of these exercises and movements include the upward dog pose, cobra pose, and extending too far on a back extension machine.

Hyperflexion means that the spine bends too far forward. This is less of a concern than hyperextension, since we commonly bend over to pull our turnout pants' suspenders over our shoulders. However, firefighters with pre-existing back injuries should avoid exercises and stretches that excessively load the spine when it is flexing. These include sit-ups, incline sit-ups, weighted ab machine, and bent-over hamstring stretches.

The side bend is a core exercise that uses lateral flexion of the spine. When executing side bends, dip your shoulder a maximum of 6 inches to the side and avoid using excessive weight.

Rule 4: Avoid Excessive Torque and Twisting of the Spine

In addition to hyperextension and hyperflexion, Dr. Moore also warns about excessive torque and twisting of the spine. In simple terms, torque is a rotational force—much like wringing out a wet rag or a baseball player swinging a bat. Low to moderate torque during core exercises is beneficial and desired. However, *excessive* torque (especially with too much weight) is detrimental because it can cause damage to the spine, vertebrae, intervertebral disks, and surrounding muscles.

Exercises that put torque on the spine are oblique twists, woodchoppers, mason twists, and standing knee-over-elbow twists. With all of these movements, make sure to go slow, choose a lower resistance, and use a medium range of motion. For example, for standing oblique twists with a cable machine (or an elastic band), twist the core approximately 120 degrees. Using a clock as a reference, this would be the equivalent of twisting your upper body from the 10 o'clock hour to the 2 o'clock hour. Overall, we definitely want to avoid going beyond 180 degrees for rotational core exercises.

Part 2: Top 10 Exercises to Improve Core Strength

The "standard" abdominal exercises of the past were the sit-up and the crunch. These exercises were ideal for carving out a set of washboard abs; however, performing these two exercises alone will not target all of the core.

When we exercise our core, we need to be universal in our approach. Therefore, exercises in a core workout should target the front, back, and sides of the torso.

When performing any core exercise, remember the four guidelines mentioned above:

1. Engage your core muscles.
2. Move slowly and in a controlled fashion.
3. Avoid hyperextension and hyperflexion of the spine.
4. Avoid excessive torque and twisting of the spine.

Listed below are 10 core exercises that range from *Level 1* (beginner) to *Level 3* (advanced). It should be mentioned that there are hundreds of core exercises. For more core exercises, visit FirefighterFunctionalFitness.com.

Level 1 contains core exercises that build stability and muscular endurance. If you are just starting to build core strength, hold each of these exercises for 10 to 20 seconds at a time. As you progress, aim to hold them for a total of 45 to 60 seconds each. Repeat these exercises in a circuit fashion for a total of two to four sets.

After you have become proficient with *Level 1* core exercises, start to incorporate those from *Level 2*.

Level 2 has exercises that also target the oblique muscles, integrate dynamic movement, and provide more of a challenge. When doing *Side Bends*, start without weight and remember to not dip your shoulder further than 6 inches (perform 10 repetitions for each side). For the *Standing Oblique Twist*, choose a low resistance at first and avoid twisting more than 120 degrees. For the *Modified Superman*, make sure your head and neck stay in line with your upper body (i.e. avoid flexing it too far upward). For the *Downward Dog*, your body should look like an upside down "V." Try to get your biceps close to your ears and your heels all the way to the ground. Hold this position for 10 to 20 seconds at first, eventually progressing to 45 to 60 seconds.

Level 3 exercises can be quite the challenge since they require optimal stability as well as muscular endurance and strength. You can start by performing the *Supine Leg Raise* for 5 to 10 repetitions (eventually building up to 15 to 20 repetitions). If you want more of a challenge, move on to a *Hanging Leg Raise* from a pull-up bar. The *Crocodile Pose* will challenge your core strength *and* upper-body strength. Start by holding it for 10 seconds and eventually build up to 30 to 60 seconds. Lastly, the *Hollow Rock* is like a human see-saw because the legs and arms go up and down in an alternating fashion. While fully engaging the core, start by rocking for 10 seconds and eventually build up to 45 to 60 seconds.

When incorporating Level 3 exercises, you can still use Levels 1 and 2, and make them more challenging by increasing hold times, repetitions, and sets. Level 3 core exercises should only be integrated after you have become proficient in Levels 1 and 2.

LEVEL 1 CORE EXERCISES

1) Standard Plank

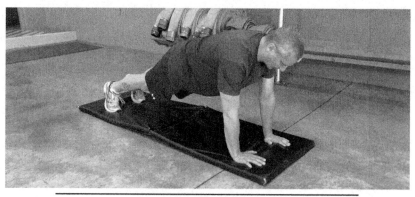

Maintain a straight line through the head, neck, back, hips, and legs.
Maintain full-body tension.

> **Progressions**: Feet elevated on bench or in suspension straps (TRX®), weight on back, lift and hold single leg and arm, lift and hold opposite arm and leg simultaneously
> **Regressions**: Forearm plank, knees on ground

2) Straight-arm Side Plank

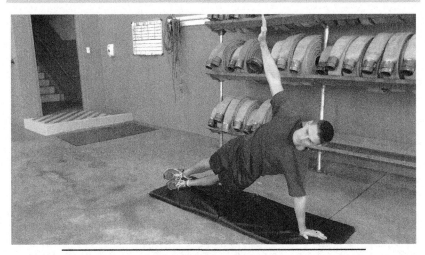

Maintain a straight line through the head, neck back, hips, and legs.
Maintain full-body tension.

> **Progressions**: Feet elevated on bench or in suspension
> straps, twist torso downward and touch ground, lift top leg,
> touch top elbow and knee together
> **Regressions**: Elbow side plank, knees on ground, top leg
> foot touching ground in front for support

3) Bridge Pose

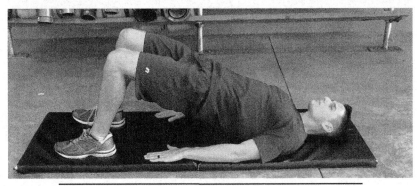

Maintain straight line from knees to shoulders; avoid sagging of hips.

> **Progressions**: Single-leg bridge pose, alternating feet
> touching the ground (marching), hold weight above body
> with both hands straight up
> **Regressions**: None

LEVEL 2 CORE EXERCISES

4) Side Bend

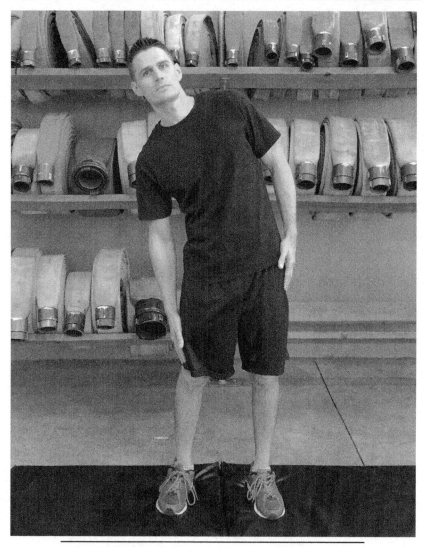

Bend 6 inches off-center and return to neutral position,
avoid excessive lateral extension.

> **Progressions**: Weighted side bend, side bend while balancing on one leg
> **Regressions**: None

5) Standing Oblique Twist

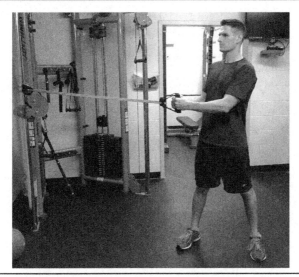

Starting position: Feet shoulder-width apart.

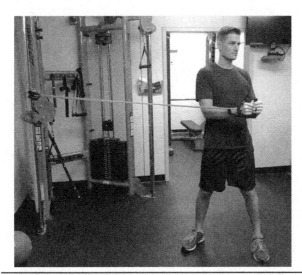

Ending position: Rotate 120 degrees, avoid excessive twisting of spine.

> **Progressions**: Increase weight or resistance, fully extend arms at end of movement

> **Regressions**: Perform without weight or resistance

6) Modified Superman

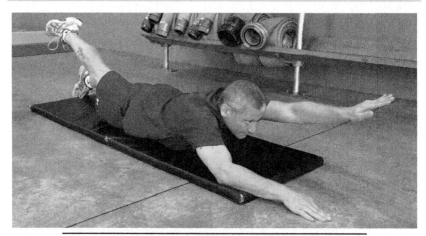

While lying prone, lift opposite leg and arm off of floor and hold.
Keep head and neck in neutral position, looking forward.

› **Progressions**: Lift all legs and arms off of ground and hold

› **Regressions**: Lift only one leg or arm off of ground at a time

7) Downward Dog

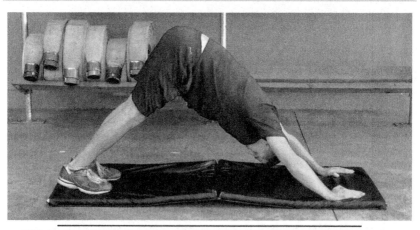

With feet and hands touching the floor, hinge at the hips while pushing the
shoulders back towards the feet to obtain an "inverted V" position.

› **Progressions**: Raise single leg or arm off of floor and hold,
elbows and forearms touching floor (instead of hands)

› **Regressions**: Bend knees to decrease intensity of leg
stretch

LEVEL 3 CORE EXERCISES

8) Supine Leg Raise

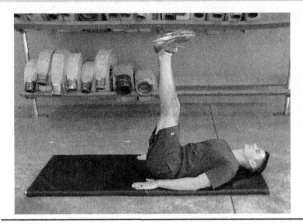

With arms, torso, and head against the floor,
lift feet to 90 degree position off of floor (keeping legs straight).

> **Progressions**: Lower legs and hold 6 inches above ground, hold stability ball in between feet (lower and raise), raise hands from overhead to touch feet at maximum extension, hanging leg raises (from pull-up bar)
> **Regressions**: Single-leg raises, raise opposite leg and arm to touch each other at maximum extension

9) Crocodile Pose

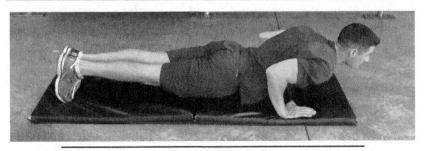

Starting in a plank position, slowly lower torso *forward* and downward,
keeping the elbows at your sides. Elbows are bent at 90-degrees.
Maintain full-body tension.

> **Progressions**: Lift and hold single leg off of floor, single-arm
> **Regressions**: Knees on ground

61

10) Hollow Rock

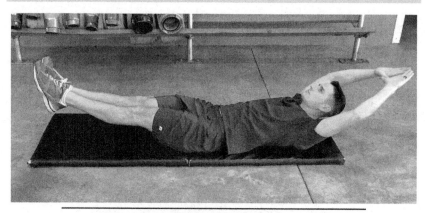

While lying supine, extend arms above head.
Use momentum to rock back and forth while keeping the core engaged.
Maintain full-body tension.

> **Progressions**: Hold light weights in hands
> **Regressions**: Instead of rocking, alternate lifting legs and then upper body off of floor while lying supine

Part 3: 6 Steps to Optimizing Core Workouts

Creating an effective core workout is vitally important and very easy to do.

Step 1. Choose to perform a core workout as a stand-alone workout or incorporate it with cardiovascular capacity training, strength training, or flexibility training. Note: a core workout can be performed immediately before or after we complete these workouts.

Step 2. Combine 3 to 10 core exercises into a circuit. Don't limit yourself to the exercises that were presented in this section. Visit FirefighterFunctionalFitness.com to expand your core exercise library.

Step 3. Pick exercises and movements that will target *all* of the core. This includes the front, back, and sides of the torso. If you know that you have an underdeveloped core and are just beginning to strengthen it, consider performing only one round of your chosen circuit. As you progress, complete the same core circuit a total of two to four rounds. An independent core workout lasting 15 to 30 minutes is a good goal to achieve.

Step 4. Strive to perform each movement for 45 to 60 seconds at a time. If you can only perform a movement for 10 seconds before fatigue sets in, only do it for 10 seconds. The next workout session that you choose to do the same movement, try to perform it for a longer duration (e.g. 20 seconds).

Step 5. Transition between each core exercise in a slow, purposeful, and controlled manner. *Remember: Core workouts are not about speed. They are about proper form and building muscular endurance.* Improper form can lead to injury, poor muscle memory, and faster onset to fatigue.

Step 6. Perform core workouts two to four times per week, even if they are initially 5 to 10 minutes per session. It is best to perform core workouts on nonconsecutive days so that your core has sufficient time to rest and recover.

Safety note: As with any exercise or movement, if anything hurts while performing a core exercise, immediately stop the movement. Consult with a certified personal trainer or physician, if necessary.

ACTION STEPS:

1. Evaluate your current core workouts. Do they focus on just "abs," or do they integrate the *entire* core?

2. Use The Big 8 to structure your core workouts. Use the top 10 core exercises presented in this chapter and their levels of difficulty.

3. Perform core strength training two to four times per week.

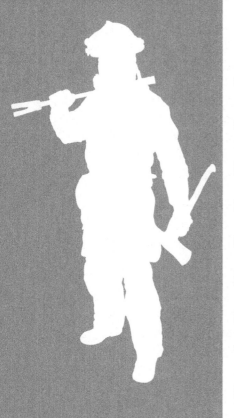

The extent to which a firefighter develops their cardiovascular capacity will ultimately determine whether they are an asset or a liability on the fireground.

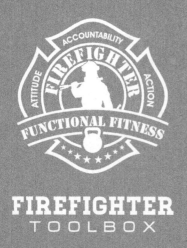

FIREFIGHTER
TOOLBOX

CHAPTER 5

THE BIG 8: CARDIOVASCULAR CAPACITY

WHAT IS CARDIOVASCULAR CAPACITY?

Within our bodies, our cardiovascular system transports oxygen from our lungs to all tissues that require oxygen. After these tissues have used enough oxygen, our blood takes metabolic byproducts (e.g. carbon dioxide) back to the lungs where they are exhaled. When performing physical activity, our bodies make adjustments to the cardiovascular system like increasing heart rate, how much blood is pumped out of the heart, and dilating blood vessels to meet the metabolic demands imposed on it.

As it pertains to *Firefighter Functional Fitness*, **cardiovascular capacity** is a combination of **cardiovascular** fitness and aerobic *capacity*. In simple terms, it is the measure of the body's *effectiveness* in transporting oxygen to working muscles and how *efficiently* these muscles exchange and use this oxygen.

Based on the physical activities that firefighters perform, optimal cardiovascular capacity is a cornerstone of our functional fitness. We could perform strength training seven days of the week and end up with a great physique, but if we do not adequately develop our cardiovascular capacity, we will not be able to perform at elite levels on the fireground.

This section is dedicated to teaching you why cardiovascular capacity is vitally important and how to properly develop it as a firefighter for optimal fireground performance.

WHY IS CARDIOVASCULAR CAPACITY IMPORTANT FOR FIREFIGHTERS?

We have all witnessed the "rehab firefighter phenomenon" before: Those firefighters who work on the fireground for 5 minutes and then they spend the next 30 minutes in the rehab sector "recovering." Their lack of performance and cardiovascular capacity is obvious to everyone.

On the other hand, firefighters with excellent cardiovascular capacity are able to perform more work, more efficiently, with less need for rest. They are also able to take shorter rest periods before getting back to firefighting activities (i.e. *less time in rehab, more time fighting fire*).

No one can deny the incredible amount of cardiovascular capacity that is required of our profession. Studies have demonstrated that we as firefighters meet or exceed our theoretical maximum heart rates when working on the fireground. Furthermore, our heart rate may stay at near-maximum for hours after a strenuous call due to the continuous release of endorphins.

Consider all of the fireground activities that require optimal cardiovascular capacity:

> Wearing and moving with full PPE (turnout gear, helmet, SCBA cylinder and mask, radio, tools, etc.)
> Forcible entry and egress
> Carrying, raising, and climbing ladders
> Stretching and advancing hose lines
> Ventilation
> Opening fire hydrants
> Search operations
> Victim and firefighter rescue
> Dragging, lifting, hoisting, and carrying heavy equipment
> Breaching walls
> Ascending stairs
> Overhaul
> Crawling, pushing, pulling, and prying

When combined with firefighter PPE and thermal stress, the activities mentioned above put incredible stress on the cardio-vascular system. There are numerous factors that contribute to the cardiovascular strain of firefighting[1]:

> **Individual health characteristics** (health status, fitness profile, family history)

> **Physical work** (wearing PPE, performing fireground tasks)

> **Heat stress and dehydration** (PPE, environmental, metabolic work)

> **Sympathetic nervous system activation** (internal endorphin release caused by alarm dispatch and dangerous/chaotic scene)

All of these factors work in conjunction to increase heart rate, the heart's stroke volume, and oxygen consumption (i.e. *cardiac workload*). In other words, the fireground causes a firefighter's heart to "work overtime" to be able to meet the incredible cardiovascular and metabolic demands that are placed on it. Unfortunately, if a firefighter lacks sufficient cardiovascular capacity, the consequences can be life-altering or even fatal.

We all would agree the job is physically demanding, but exactly how hard do we work at a fire scene? Fortunately, specific aspects of a firefighter's workload have been measured and quantified.

A MET (Metabolic Equivalent of a Task) is the rate of oxygen consumption during a task (as compared to resting). VO_2 (Volume of Oxygen) is another measurement of oxygen consumption that is typically used. Resting carries a MET value of 1, whereas running on a treadmill at 6.5 mph is equivalent to 10.7 METS. *All of the firefighting activities listed below have greater oxygen and metabolic demands than running at a speed of 6.5 mph.*

Research has demonstrated the following MET and VO_2 values for common firefighting activities:

> **Ascending stairs with turnout gear and SCBA =** 11 METS or VO_2 value of 39 mL/(kg•min)

> **Carrying tools up stairs with turnout gear & SCBA =** 12.5 METS or VO_2 value of 44 mL/(kg•min)

> **Search and rescue of victims under smoke conditions =** 16 METS or VO_2 of 56 mL/(kg•min)

These MET/VO_2 values are very similar to those of professional athletes who play football, basketball, soccer, etc. But how many firefighters do you know who are physically fit enough to achieve and *maintain* these values for the duration of a fire? Unfortunately, the most likely answer is: *Not that many.*

According to the National Fire Protection Association Standard 1582: *Standard on Comprehensive Occupational Medical Program for Fire Departments*, firefighters must achieve a minimum VO_2 value of 42 mL/(kg•min) to safely perform firefighting tasks.

Take a moment of honest introspection to ask yourself if you are functionally fit to fight fire. If the answer is "no," what changes need to be made for you to achieve your optimal cardiovascular capacity? If you are unsure, then *Firefighter Functional Fitness* will be your guide on how to optimize your performance and thrive on the fireground.

HOW TO IMPROVE FIREFIGHTER CARDIOVASCULAR CAPACITY

We can improve cardiovascular capacity through frequent physical exercise—that which will consistently elevate and sustain our heart rate. By frequently increasing our cardiac output, we improve our heart and lungs' metabolic capacity, blood plasma volume, and muscular endurance.

Improving cardiorespiratory capacity through frequent exercise will lead to:

> ➤ Improved capacity to perform work
> ➤ Improved endurance, stamina, and resiliency
> ➤ Shortened recovery and rest periods
> ➤ Reduction in fatigue
> ➤ Reduced incidence of dehydration
> ➤ Reduction in risk of injury
> ➤ Reduction in risk of heart attack and cardiovascular disease

> Reduction of risk of sudden cardiac death from firefighting duties
> Positive effects on blood pressure, weight, cholesterol, blood glucose, mood, and more

For functionally fit firefighters, there are two primary ways to improve cardiovascular capacity:

1. **High-intensity interval training**
2. **Endurance-based cardiovascular training**

Both of these methods are extremely important and applicable to our functional fitness as firefighters.

Before we examine these two methods, please refer to the following chart to obtain your maximum heart rate, your target heart rate for high-intensity interval training (HIIT), and your target heart rate for endurance-based cardiovascular training (EBCT).

Table 5.1 – HEART RATE CHART			
AGE	**70% Target HR EBCT**	**85% Target HR HIIT**	**MAXIMUM HEART RATE**
20	140	170	200
25	137	166	195
30	133	162	190
35	130	157	185
40	126	153	180
45	123	149	175
50	119	145	170
55	116	140	165
60	112	136	160
65	109	132	155
70	105	128	150

To calculate your estimated maximum heart rate, use the following formula:

220 Beats Per Minute – Age = Maximum Heart Rate (MHR)

HIGH-INTENSITY INTERVAL TRAINING

High-intensity interval training (HIIT) combines alternating periods of vigorous exercise with recovery periods of lesser intensity. These intervals should be repeated for a total duration of 20 to 60 minutes per workout. HIIT improves explosive cardiovascular capacity and shortens recovery periods by attaining your near-maximal heart rate.

The high-intensity period can last anywhere from 15 seconds to more than 5 minutes in duration. The recovery period should last the same amount of time or less. The overall goal is to increase the high-intensity activity duration and shorten the recovery period. For example, an excellent goal would be to perform 3 to 5 minutes of continuous high-intensity training, followed by a 1 minute recovery period. However, for deconditioned ("out of shape") firefighters who want to start HIIT, 10 to 30 seconds of high-intensity with 1 to 3 minutes of recovery is entirely appropriate. As always, listen to your body and start small.

There are several fireground tasks that are representative of HIIT:

> - Stretching and advancing hose lines
> - Forcible entry or egress
> - Roof and window ventilation
> - Carrying, raising, and climbing ladders
> - Search and rescue of a civilian or firefighter
> - Carrying, dragging, and crawling with heavy equipment
> - Ascending stairs

All of these tasks require intense bursts of cardiovascular capacity to meet the body's metabolic demands. They are then usually followed by a brief "recovery" period where a firefighter engages in less intense physical activity.

Not only is HIIT excellent for developing our cardiovascular capacity, but it is also highly effective for losing weight. The National Academy of Sports Medicine (NASM) states that HIIT is superior to moderate-intensity, long-duration exercise because it burns more calories and subcutaneous fat, as well as boosting post-workout metabolism levels[2].

HOW TO INCORPORATE HIIT INTO WORKOUTS

When using HIIT in our workouts, our goal is to elevate our heart rate to 85 to 95 percent of our maximum heart rate during the high-intensity periods. To calculate your HIIT target heart rate, take your maximum heart rate and multiply it by 0.85 to 0.95. For example, a 40-year old will have a HIIT target heart rate between 153 BPM to 171 BPM (Calculation: 180 BPM x 0.85 = 153 BPM OR 180 BPM x 0.95 = 171 BPM). For simplicity's sake, we could average the HIIT target heart rate at 162 BPM for a 40-year old firefighter.

If you do not have the ability to monitor your heart rate during HIIT, you can simply monitor your respiratory rate. For example, if you are breathing hard enough that you can only speak in one or two-word phrases, you have reached a suitable HIIT activity level. However, to obtain the most accurate heart rate readings, we recommend using a personal heart rate monitor (e.g. Polar® chest strap and/or watch).

Incorporating HIIT into exercise sessions is very simple. Refer to the following tables for some examples of conventional HIIT exercises, as well as firefighter-specific HIIT exercises.

Table 5.2 – CONVENTIONAL HIIT EXERCISES	
1	Sprinting
2	Running Stairs, Step-mill, Stair Climber
3	Swimming
4	Stationary Bike
5	Row Machine
6	Boxing/Punching Bag
7	Jumping Rope
8	Battle Ropes
9	Plyometrics (box jumps, squat jumps, tuck jumps)
10	Strength-training circuits (bodyweight exercises, dumbbells/weights, kettlebells, etc.)

* With any of these exercises, give near-maximal effort for the high-intensity phase and then back off to minimal effort for the recovery

periods. Using the treadmill as example, a functionally fit firefighter could theoretically sprint at 8 to 9 mph for 1 minute, and then jog leisurely at 4 to 5 mph during their recovery period. On the other hand, a deconditioned firefighter might run at 6 mph for 30 seconds, and then walk at 3 mph for 2 minutes during their recovery period.

Table 5.3 – FIREFIGHTER-SPECIFIC HIIT EXERCISE LIST	
1	Stair Climber or Ascending Stairs
2	Jacobs Ladder
3	Ground Ladder or Aerial Ladder Climb
4	Ladder Carry and Raise
5	Firefighter Crawl
6	Forcible Entry Simulator
7	Sledgehammer Tire Strike
8	Heavy Equipment Carry
9	Battle Hose
10	Pulling Ceiling Simulation
11	Pulling Charged Hose Line Simulation
12	Equipment Rope Hoist
13	Hose Line Crawl
14	Hose Line Bear Crawl

Any of the above activities can be used for HIIT. There is virtually no limit to the variety of HIIT exercises that can be performed. When performing HIIT, find the appropriate balance of performing at near-maximum effort while not overexerting yourself to the point of complete exhaustion. If you cannot maintain proper form while executing a movement, slow down or stop the exercise.

One of the ultimate ways to improve firefighter functional fitness through HIIT is to combine several of firefighting activities (listed above) into a training circuit. Put on your helmet, boots, gloves, and turnout gear and then perform each task for 20 to 60 seconds of high intensity. Then move to the next station in the circuit.

Here is an example of a HIIT circuit:

1. Stair climb (two flights)
2. Equipment hoist and lower (25 feet up and down, 50 pounds attached to a rope)
3. Sledgehammer tire strike (10 strikes with each arm leading, 20 total)
4. Ground ladder carry, raise, and climb (24-foot ladder)
5. Charged hose line crawl and pull (crawl 25 feet with the nozzle, pull remaining 25 feet towards you)

Repeat this circuit two to five times, depending on your current fitness level. It is acceptable for beginners to perform this firefighter circuit training for a total of 10 minutes wearing just gym clothes.

As our fitness level improves, we can increase the level of difficulty by donning turnout gear, and eventually start to add additional firefighting accessories (helmet, SCBA cylinder/mask, radio, flashlight, etc.). For the functionally fit firefighter, the goal is to wear all fireground PPE, mask-up, and go "on-air" for the entire workout. Lastly, the *ultimate challenge* would be to continuously repeat the circuit to see how long we can make the air in our SCBA cylinders last.

HIIT AND STRENGTH TRAINING: WHY SHOULD FIREFIGHTERS COMBINE THEM?

The overarching goals of HIIT are to improve work performance, explosive cardiovascular capacity, and recovery in a manner that supports and represents firefighter performance and function (i.e. short bursts of high-intensity, strength-based work).

If we really want to break down fireground physical activities into a form of workout, they are basically a combination of HIIT and strength training. Therefore, any workout that safely and effectively combines these two elements will drastically improve our functional fitness.

There are several established exercise methods and programs that blend HIIT and strength training:

> CrossFit®
> Tabata (8 rounds of 20-seconds on, 10-seconds rest = 4 minutes total)
> Insanity®
> P90X®
> Strength circuit training with weights, kettlebells, and bodyweight exercises
> Fitness "boot camps"

We do not endorse any single method over the others. What we do want to emphasize is to make sure that your chosen method of HIIT closely resembles the movements, techniques, intensity, and dynamic fitness of the fireground. Furthermore, the exercise equipment and method(s) you choose should always be performed properly, safely, and with good form.

When performing any exercise, ask yourself these three questions: 1) Is it *safe*? 2) Is it *effective*? 3) Is it *functional*?"

Remember: Correct form and body mechanics are always more important than how fast an exercise can be completed or how much weight is used. Utilizing proper form and function will reduce risk of injury and rate of fatigue.

ENDURANCE-BASED CARDIOVASCULAR TRAINING

We often say our time in the fire service is a marathon, not a sprint. In the same vein, we must possess a high level of *cardiovascular endurance* to perform the marathon of firefighting tasks during a working fire.

HIIT will give us the explosive cardiovascular capacity required for short periods of intense activity on the fireground. On the other hand, **endurance-based cardiovascular training** (EBCT) will round out cardiovascular capacity to ensure that we have optimal *stamina* and *endurance,* while simultaneously reducing rates and levels of fatigue.

EBCT is very straightforward: Perform moderate-intensity physical activity that will sustain your heart rate at 70 percent of your maximum heart rate. If you cannot monitor your heart rate, make sure that the exercise that you are performing is elevating your respiratory rate substantially. However, you should still have enough breath to speak in full sentences (unlike HIIT).

Make it a goal to perform this type of training for 30 to 60 minutes within a single workout.

To calculate your target heart rate for this type of exercise, take your maximum heart rate and multiply it by 0.7. For example, a 40-year old will have a target heart rate of 126 BPM for endurance-based cardiovascular training (Calculation: 180 BPM x 0.7 = 126 BPM).

Conventional physical activities like running, swimming, biking, step mill, rowing, elliptical trainer, etc., are all suitable avenues for this type of cardiovascular training. However, to make endurance-based cardiovascular training more *functional,* don a set of turnout gear and perform moderate-intensity firefighting activities: walking, crawling, climbing ladders, carrying equipment, walking up and down stairs, etc.

For more of a challenge, grab additional firefighting accessories like your helmet, SCBA mask and cylinder, radio, and a tool to carry. Again, the last step to making this type of exercise even more functional is to mask-up and breathe while using the SCBA.

HOW MUCH CARDIOVASCULAR TRAINING IS ENOUGH?

The American College of Sports Medicine has made the following recommendation on the quality and quantity of weekly exercise: The general adult population should perform *at least* 150 minutes of moderate-intensity exercise (e.g. fast walk, light jog, etc.) or 75 minutes of vigorous-intensity exercise (e.g. HIIT, EBCT, strength training, etc.) every week. These figures are where health benefits *start* to present themselves.

As firefighters, however, we know that the physical nature of our profession requires substantially more from us than that of the general population. Therefore, our amount of weekly exercise should well exceed the aforementioned numbers. *Functionally fit firefighters should strive for 300 minutes of moderate-intensity exercise or 150 minutes of vigorous-intensity exercise every week.* To simplify, we can break this up into vigorous 30-minute workouts, five days per week.

> ❝ Functionally fit firefighters should strive for 300 minutes of moderate-intensity exercise or 150 minutes of vigorous-intensity exercise every week."

These figures may seem like a lot, but remember that any moderate to vigorous physical exercise can fit under these categories, as long as our heart rate is in a suitable range. For example, conventional strength training, yoga, and a core-strengthening circuit are suitable alternatives to running or using the stair climber—provided that we maintain a heart rate of 70 percent of our maximum heart rate.

Throughout the week or even in the same workout, it is perfectly acceptable to combine EBCT and HIIT. Again, our primary goal is to prepare our bodies for realistic fireground performance. Whatever you choose to implement as cardiovascular capacity training is completely up to you. Be creative, keep it interesting, and do what you enjoy.

Lastly, when thinking about importance of cardiovascular training and how it relates to the health and safety of firefighters, consider this: studies show that regular aerobic exercise can reduce the risk of heart attack by 50 percent or more. Therefore, improving our cardiovascular capacity lays a solid foundation not only for firefighter functional fitness but also for our general health and safety.

ACTION STEPS:

1. Know the difference between high-intensity interval training (HIIT) and endurance-based cardiovascular training (EBCT). Know why each is vitally important to your functional fitness.

2. Calculate and memorize your maximum heart rate using this formula: 220 - AGE = MHR.

3. Calculate and memorize your HIIT heart rate (MHR x 0.85) and your EBCT heart rate (MHR x 0.70). Use these numbers as benchmarks during your cardiovascular capacity workouts.

4. For workouts that are aimed to improve cardiovascular capacity, incorporate at least one HIIT session *and* one EBCT session per week. Choose exercises that you enjoy doing. You don't have do the same exercise or machine for the entire 30-minute duration. It is actually more beneficial to incorporate multiple activities in a circuit training format to work multiple areas of your body.

5. Do one firefighter-specific circuit training session per week. Get creative with the fireground activities that you choose for each session. With each passing week, challenge yourself to add three to five minutes to each session.

6. Check out FirefighterFunctionalFitness.com for more great cardiovascular capacity workout ideas.

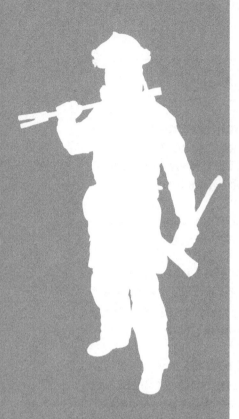

Functionally fit firefighters are able to bend without breaking.

This is the very essence of flexibility.

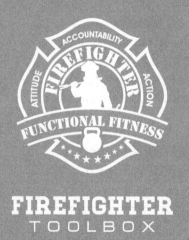

FIREFIGHTER
TOOLBOX

CHAPTER 6

THE BIG 8: FLEXIBILITY

WHAT IS FLEXIBILITY?

Flexibility is the ability of a muscle and joint to move through a full range of motion. The capacity of a joint to move through its full range of motion is dependent on the surrounding tissues and their ability to elongate. Flexibility is an essential component of our overall mobility, performance, and functional fitness as firefighters.

WHY IS FLEXIBILITY IMPORTANT FOR FIREFIGHTERS?

Sprains, strains, and back injuries are the leading injuries for firefighters. There are more than 1 million firefighters in the United States; 44 percent of these firefighters have sustained a sprain or strain injury while on duty[3].

A lack of flexibility (and lack of core strength) not only leads to an increased risk of these injuries but also to an increase in their severity, recovery duration, employer and employee costs, and lost time. Furthermore, a lack of flexibility decreases mobility, which is especially important since a firefighter's protective ensemble already restricts range of motion. Functionally fit firefighters understand the importance of flexibility as part of a well-rounded fitness program, and they apply good stretching techniques to their workout regimens.

There are several other benefits to regular flexibility training:

> - Improves muscular strength, endurance, power, and recovery
> - Improves cardiovascular capacity and physical performance
> - Reduces the severity and duration of muscle fatigue and soreness
> - Increases mental and physical relaxation
> - Improves balance, stability, and posture
> - Improves your ability to perform exercises with correct form

Similar to many other aspects of firefighter fitness, the average firefighter does not place enough importance on flexibility training. Additionally, long sedentary periods (e.g. sitting too long, "recliner time," etc.) only compound the problem—especially when we have the potential to go from a deep sleep to a chaotic fireground in only a matter of minutes.

We cannot eliminate or avoid all line-of-duty injuries, just like we cannot prevent all LODDs. However, functionally fit firefighters understand that we can significantly manage our risks by incorporating regular flexibility training into our fitness routines. Doing so will not only reduce the risk and incidence of injuries, it will also improve our fireground performance.

HOW TO IMPROVE FLEXIBILITY

We will focus on three primary concepts that improve flexibility:

1. Stretching exercises
2. Functional yoga
3. Cardiovascular capacity training

Within this chapter, we will dedicate our time to discussing *stretching exercises* and *functional yoga*. For more information on how cardiovascular capacity training impacts our flexibility, please refer to Chapter 5 *The Big 8: Cardiovascular Capacity*.

Firefighter Functional Fitness primarily uses two types of stretching: *static* and *dynamic*.

Static stretching typically involves a single joint through a simple movement which is *held* in a stationary manner. Static stretches are held for at least 30 seconds and are to be used *after* the muscles and joints are completely warmed up. They are used during cool-down routines (after the conditioning phase of a workout) and during functional yoga sessions.

Examples of static stretches include holding a butterfly (groin) stretch, runner's lunge, and medial arm stretch. The medial arm stretch is pictured below.

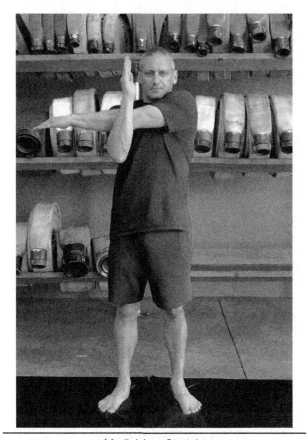

Medial Arm Stretch.

Dynamic stretching involves a joint's full or near-full range of motion while one set of muscles lengthen and an opposite set of muscles contract. In simple terms, dynamic stretching incorporates stretching and stability while the body is *in motion*. This type of stretching will use a constant series of movements to progressively lengthen the target muscles.

Dynamic stretching is ideal during warm-ups to prepare the body for the conditioning phase of a workout. Exercises that use dynamic stretching include air squats, lunges, and arm circles. In all of these movements, the body is *in motion*, progressively stretching the muscles. Using lunges as a dynamic stretch is pictured below.

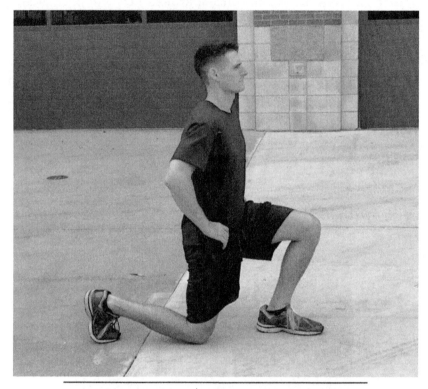

Lunges.

HOW IMPORTANT IS IT TO STRETCH BEFORE OR AFTER EXERCISING?

There has been much debate about whether or not to stretch before or after the conditioning phase of our workouts. In the past, some of us may have been taught to stretch immediately before we engage in exercise. However, research has shown that "cold stretching" (i.e.

static stretching without a warm-up) before strength training has actually decreased muscular power[4].

It is always better to perform a brief warm-up before any kind of static stretching (and before every exercise session). This translates to performing 5 to 10 minutes of foam rolling of tight muscles, brisk walking, jogging, step mill, and even using *dynamic stretching*. For example, if we are going to exercise our lower body, we will use air squats, lunges, and tube-walking with an elastic band as our preparatory dynamic stretches. Completing a warm-up will increase muscular blood flow, body temperature, range of motion, and muscular pliability.

Immediately following cardiovascular capacity and strength training sessions, we will perform 5 to 10 minutes of flexibility training. For the post-workout cool-down, we will use static stretching. Doing so will decrease muscle soreness and improve recovery.

DISCOMFORT VS. PAIN

While performing stretching movements, it is normal to feel mild to moderate *discomfort*; however, it is not normal to feel actual *pain* during a stretch. If you do, return to a slower pace or decreased range of movement until the pain subsides. Remember, our overall goal is to lengthen and loosen muscles by slowly and cautiously overloading the muscle—*not to induce pain*.

GUIDELINES TO PROPER STRETCHING: DURATION, FREQUENCY, AND TIPS

1. Warm up with 5 minutes of foam rolling, brisk walking, jogging, biking, etc. before any type of stretching. After warming up your muscles, continue to warm up using dynamic stretches that closely relate to the imminent workout.
2. After the conditioning phase of your workout, perform static stretches during the cool-down phase that apply to the joints and muscle groups that you just used.
3. Take your time, relax, and breathe normally when stretching. When you exhale, sink a little deeper into each stretch.

4. Hold each static stretch for at least 30 seconds and repeat each stretch for a total of two to three rounds.

5. Stretch to mild or moderate discomfort, but not to pain. Stretch slowly and cautiously to loosen joints and lengthen muscles.

6. Stretch at least three to four times a week. Stretch before and after workouts and also complete a stand-alone flexibility training session (e.g. functional yoga).

STRETCHES, POSES, AND MOVEMENTS FOR FLEXIBILITY TRAINING

Back

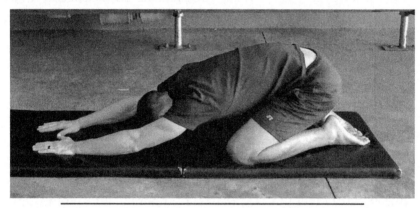

Child's Pose: While kneeling on the floor, let the torso sink down while simultaneously extending the arms overhead.

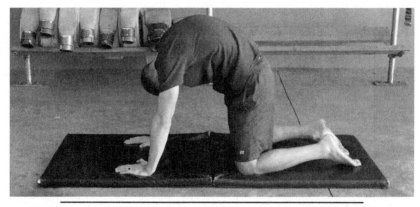

Cat Pose: Arch the back to the ceiling and hold. Alternate with Cow Pose.

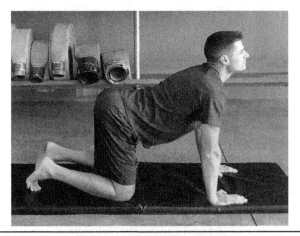

Cow pose: Arch the back downward and hold. Alternate with Cat Pose.

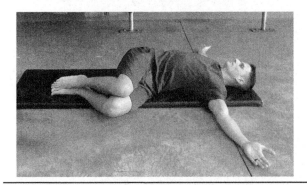

Two-knee twist: As both knees fall to the side, keep your back against the ground to avoid excessive twisting.

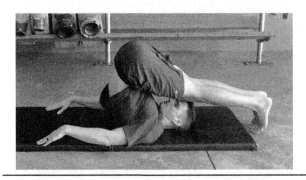

Plow pose: With shoulders planted against the ground, gently bring your feet over your head to touch the ground.

85

Core

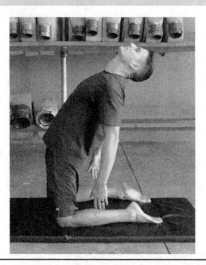

Modified-camel pose: While kneeling, gently lean backwards while engaging the core. Avoid hyperextension of the spine.

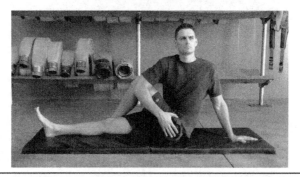

Seated Oblique twist: Gently twist the torso to stretch your obliques and hips by placing your opposite arm on the opposite leg.

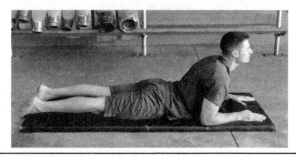

Baby-cobra pose: While lying prone, gently elevate head, shoulders, chest off of floor. Avoid hyperextension of the spine.

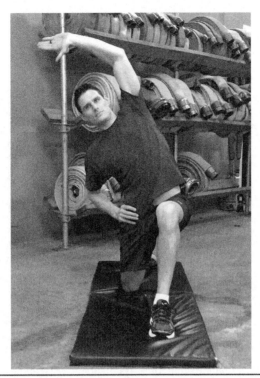

Kneeling Side Stretch: While kneeling, place one leg in front of the body. With the opposite arm, reach to the opposite side of the body.

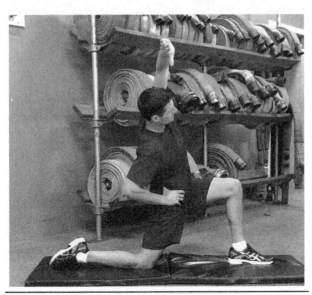

Kneeling Side Stretch: Side view.

Legs

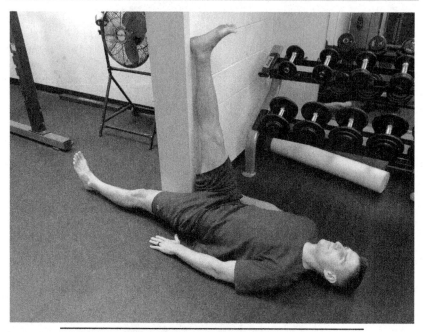

Supine hamstring wall stretch: While lying supine, raise and place leg against a wall/doorway.

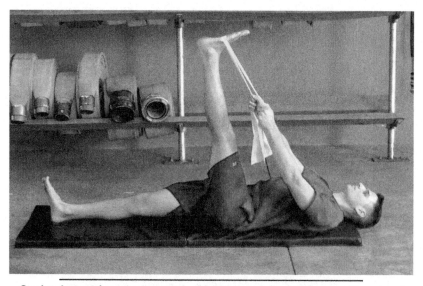

Supine hamstring strap stretch: While lying supine, raise leg with a strap/ elastic band and hold at 90 degrees.

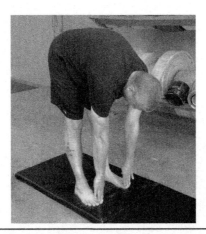

Bent-over hamstring & back stretch: From a standing position,
bend over at the hips to reach your ankles or the floor.
Do not perform if this movement hurts your back.

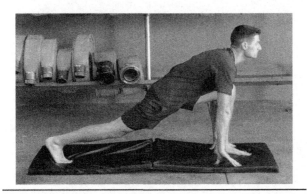

Runner's lunge: Extend the front leg in a bent position while keeping the back
leg straight.

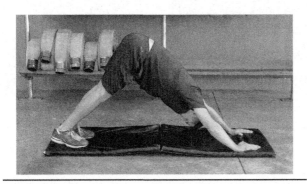

Downward dog: With feet and hands touching the floor, hinge at the hips while
pushing the shoulders back towards the feet to obtain an "inverted V" position.

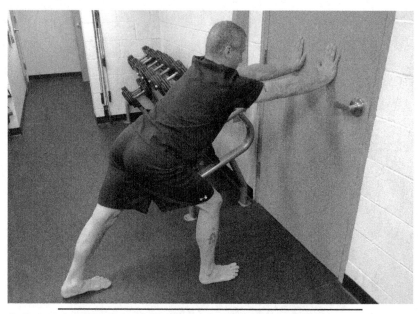

Calf stretch: While facing a wall, extend one leg behind the body and plant your foot. Lean into the wall to stretch the calf muscle.

Hip Complex

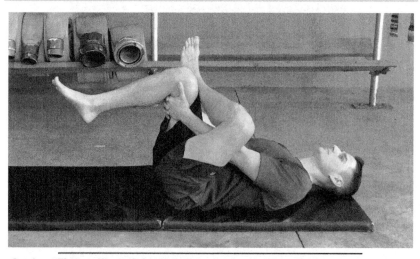

Supine "Figure 4" stretch: While lying supine, bring ankle to opposite leg and bend both knees. Pull thigh towards torso to stretch the hip.

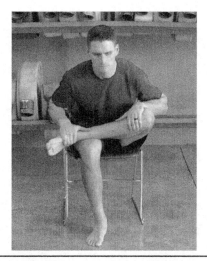

Seated "Figure 4" stretch: While seated in a chair, bring ankle to opposite leg and lean forward to stretch the hip.

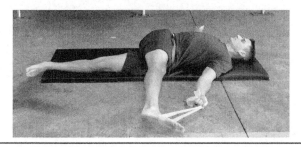

Supine hip twist with strap: While lying supine, place strap/elastic band around foot. Extend foot to opposite side of body and hold.

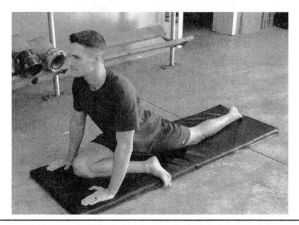

Pigeon pose: Extend bent leg in front of body to stretch the hip. For a greater stretch, lean the torso forward.

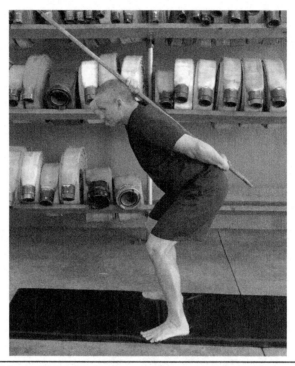

Dowel hip hinge: Stand with two arms grasping a long dowel rod/broom handle. Simultaneously bend at the hips and at the knees.

Groin

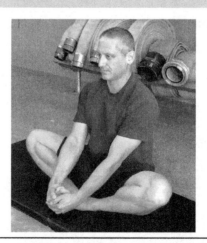

Butterfly: While sitting, touch the soles of the feet together. Pull them towards the body. Gently push the thighs downward for a greater stretch.

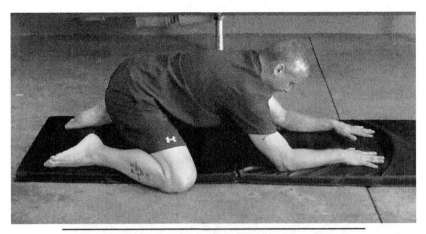

Frog pose: From a kneeling position, spread the legs apart like a frog. Sink the upper body towards the floor.

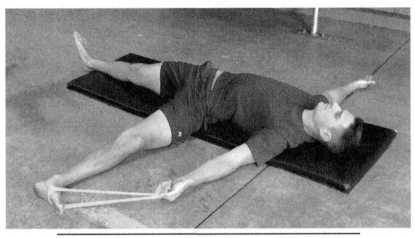

Supine groin and hip opener: While lying supine, use a strap around the foot and extend the leg laterally.

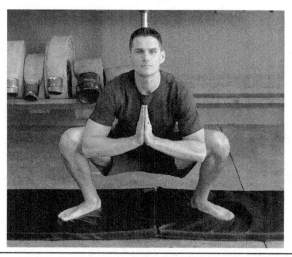

Garland pose: From a standing position, stand with feet slightly wider than shoulder-width. Sink the torso towards the floor. For a greater stretch, hold a weight with both hands.

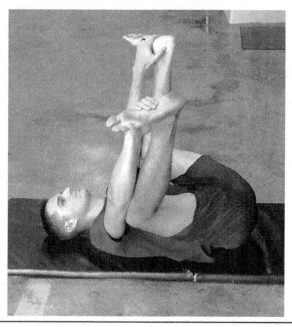

Happy baby pose: While lying supine, grab the insides of both feet with hands. Spread legs apart while pulling feet towards the floor.

Chest

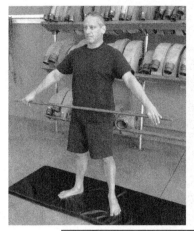 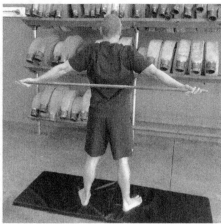

Chest opener with dowel rod: With a wide grip, grab dowel rod and extend it overhead and behind the back. Use a slow and controlled motion (starting and ending positions, rear view).

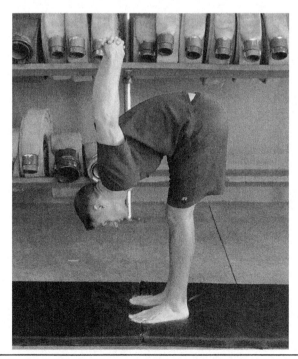

Hands together behind back: Grasp hands together behind the back. Bend over and extend hands upward.

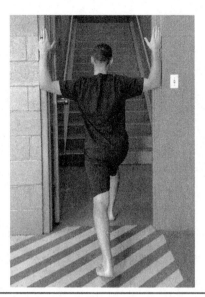

Doorway Stretch: Place both forearms against open doorway and lean forward.

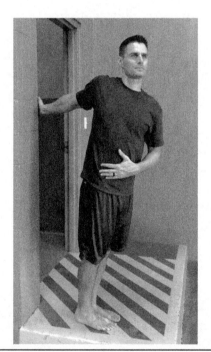

Parallel Arm Chest Stretch: Using a doorway, reach backwards with the arm. Twist away from the doorway to stretch the arm and chest.

Neck

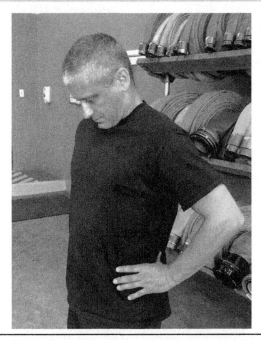

Chin to chest: Look towards the floor, stretching the posterior of the neck.

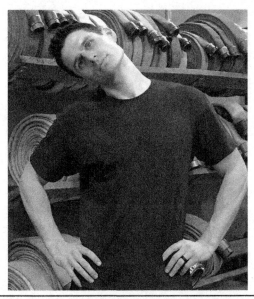

Head to Shoulder: Laterally bend head towards the shoulder. For a greater stretch, use hand on top of head to pull with gentle traction.

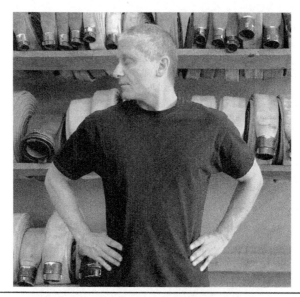

Lateral twist: Gently twist head 90 degrees.
Avoid excessive twisting/torque of neck.

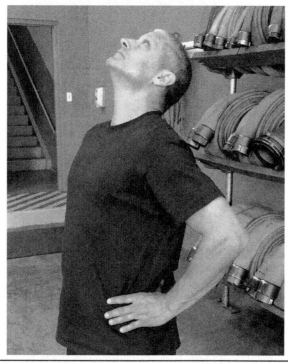

Chin pointed upwards: Bend the head back to stretch the front of the neck.

Arms and Shoulders

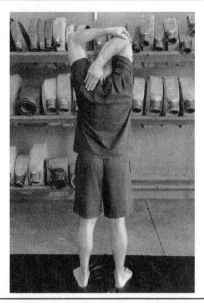

Tricep stretch: Bend elbow and reach behind head. For a greater stretch, grab elbow with opposite hand and pull with gentle traction.

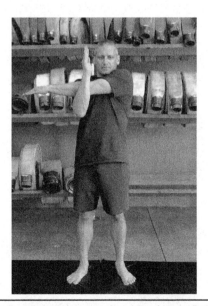

Medial arm stretch: Reach arm to opposite side of body. Pull gentle traction with non-stretching arm at the elbow.

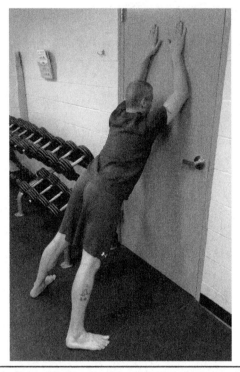

Wall stretch: Extend both arms above head and lean against the wall.

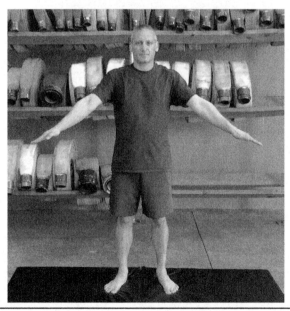

Arm circles: Extend arms laterally and rotate them in a circular motion. Use smaller circles to start and then progress to larger circles.

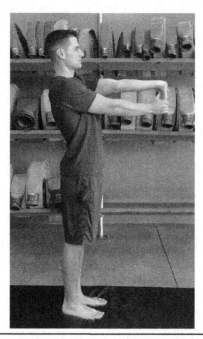

Forearm stretch: Extend arm directly in front of body. While keeping arm straight, use opposite hand to pull gentle traction on fingertips.

There are many other stretches that can be added to your flexibility training routines. The overall goal is to target *all* muscle groups. Regardless of the stretches you choose, make sure that you avoid hyperflexion, hyperextension, and excessive torque on the spine since these actions can do more damage than good. If you have a pre-existing back injury, avoid stretches that might strain on your back (e.g. bent-over hamstring stretch).

A FEW WORDS ON FUNCTIONAL YOGA

Disclaimer: *Firefighter Functional Fitness* incorporates basic yoga movements, stretches, and poses to give firefighters a balanced approach to improving their flexibility. While some yoga practices integrate spirituality and religion, *Firefighter Functional Fitness* only incorporates the *physical* aspects of yoga.

Functional yoga is an excellent medium of flexibility training because it combines basic stretches, movements, and poses in a holistic approach. We want firefighters to use it because it incorporates:

101

> Static stretching
> Dynamic stretching
> Core strength
> Strength training (muscular endurance and strength)
> Cardiovascular capacity training
> Relaxation and meditation

Unfortunately, yoga carries a negative stigma with some firefighters. These skeptics have the unfounded beliefs that yoga is "just for women" or that it will not improve their fitness. We have frequently heard firefighters say, "I can't do yoga. I'm not flexible enough." These individuals may believe that the goal of yoga is to contort oneself into unrealistic, impractical "pretzel-like" positions.

On the contrary, functional yoga is for everyone—*especially* firefighters who lack flexibility.

Table 6.1 – BENEFITS OF FUNCTIONAL YOGA [5]	
1	Increases flexibility, range of motion, and balance
2	Reduces risk of injury from sprains and strains
3	Lubricates tendons, joints, and ligaments
4	Increases muscular strength and endurance
5	Reduces stress, depression, and anxiety
6	Reduces risk factors for heart disease (weight, blood pressure, etc.)
7	Improves quality of sleep
8	Increases energy levels
9	Improves posture
10	Improves breathing
11	Decreases chronic pain (e.g. back pain)
12	Alleviate chronic health conditions (e.g. arthritis, fibromyalgia)

Unfortunately, a book is not the best medium to teach firefighters how to do functional yoga. As most would agree, it is an activity that is best-suited for live, one-on-one instruction from a trained yoga instructor. However, we have given examples of functional yoga poses that will improve flexibility and core strength. Yoga has gained enormous popularity, and classes are readily available in most areas. There are stand-alone yoga studios, and yoga is also taught at major gyms (e.g. Gold's Gym, Lifetime Fitness, 24-Hour Fitness).

For a free and simple way to practice yoga in the comfort of your firehouse or home, use your computer, tablet, or mobile device to search the Internet (or YouTube) for basic yoga instructional videos. Use the following keywords: *basic yoga workout, beginner's yoga, yoga for core strength, yoga for flexibility, power yoga,* etc.

ACTION STEPS:

1. **Use dynamic stretching during warm-ups. Use static stretching during cool-downs.**

2. **Evaluate your current workouts. Establish a journal to record your flexibility sessions. Record the dates, times, and types of stretches and poses used.**

3. **Perform flexibility training three to four times each week before and after workout sessions and as stand-alone workouts.**

4. **Use the flexibility exercises presented in this section to improve your functional fitness.**

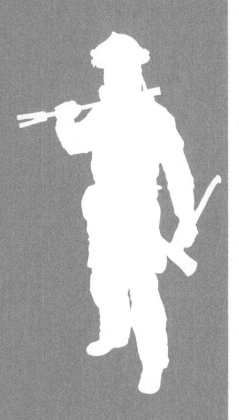

Functional strength centers around the concept of performance, not muscle mass.

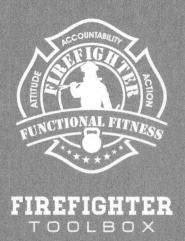

CHAPTER 7

INTRODUCTION TO FUNCTIONAL STRENGTH TRAINING

Before we move into the remaining strength-based movements of The Big 8, we will discuss the principles of functional strength training. Functionally fit firefighters know that strength training, also known as *resistance training*, is an integral part of achieving and maintaining functional fitness.

WHAT IS FUNCTIONAL STRENGTH?

In order to explain functional strength, we must understand each of the elements involved. Let's break it down into two parts:

Strength

Strength refers to the ability to exert physical force. In simple terms, to build muscular strength, endurance, and power, we have to provide the appropriate **intensity**, **volume**, and **mode** of muscular resistance.

Function

Quite simply, *function* refers to the capability of serving the natural or designed purpose. As firefighters, it is critical that we perform strength training that specifically improves on our fireground *function* and *performance* as opposed to merely "getting stronger" and "building muscle." In other words, general strength training may make us stronger and build our physique, but not all strength exercises will improve our ability to efficiently and effectively carry out firefighting tasks. The methods of strength training found in *Firefighter Functional Fitness* are specifically tailored to optimizing firefighter performance.

3 FUNDAMENTALS OF FUNCTIONAL STRENGTH

As firefighters, we perform strength training for three primary purposes: building muscular *strength*, *endurance*, and *power*. Let's explain each and describe their importance to our functional fitness.

1. **Muscular Strength**: This is the ability of a muscle or group of muscles to exert *maximum* force. Firefighters need this type of strength when operating at maximum capacity: lifting extremely heavy objects, dragging victims or firefighters, etc.

   To improve muscular strength, use heavier weights (or perform high-resistance exercises) with fewer repetitions. For example: Use 80 to 100 percent of your single-repetition maximum* for 3 to 5 sets with 1 to 8 repetitions per set. If you are at your single-rep max, you will only be able to do one repetition per set. If you are at 80 percent of your single-rep max, you will be able to do more than 1 repetition.

*To find out what your single-rep max (SRM) is for different exercises, consult with a certified personal trainer.

2. **Muscular Endurance**: This the ability of a muscle or group of muscles to exert a moderate amount of force in a very repetitious manner. Firefighters need muscular endurance to perform the marathon of firefighting tasks for the entire duration of a fire.

   To improve muscular endurance, use moderate weight (or medium-resistance exercises) with more repetitions. Therefore, 50 to 70 percent of your single-rep max for 3 to 6 sets with 8 to 20 repetitions per set. When performing isometric strength training (e.g. planks), muscular endurance is also developed by holding the position for a longer duration.

3. **Muscular Power**: This is the ability of a muscle or group of muscles to use explosive force over a minimal amount of time. Firefighters use muscular power when they strike objects: forcible entry/egress, overhaul, etc.

To improve muscular power, perform explosive movements with very high-intensity and minimal rest intervals. Power exercises include medicine ball throws, burpees, striking the Keiser Force™ machine, striking a tire with a sledgehammer/axe, kettlebell or barbell cleans, plyometrics, speed, agility, and quickness training, etc.

Let's discuss how we can build muscular strength, endurance, and power for a chest press exercise:

> ‣ To develop muscular strength, we will perform a standing cable chest press with heavy weight for 4 to 8 reps.
> ‣ To build muscular endurance, we will use the same exercise but decrease the weight to a moderate amount and perform 15 to 20 reps.
> ‣ To build muscular power, we will use a medium-weight medicine ball (15 pounds) and explosively push or throw it away from us for 10 reps.

Table 7.1 – BENEFITS OF FUNCTIONAL STRENGTH TRAINING	
1	Increased muscular strength, endurance, and power
2	Improved muscle coordination and balance
3	Increased tensile strength of tendons, ligaments, and muscles
4	Improved cardiovascular capacity, metabolism, cholesterol and hormone levels
5	Decreased body fat
6	Increased bone density

HOW TO IMPROVE FUNCTIONAL STRENGTH

Functionally fit firefighters understand that functional strength training is a process.

In order to describe this process in simple terms, we have broken it down in to four parts called the **4 R's of Strength Training: Resistance, Rest, Recovery, and Repair.**

When subjecting our muscle groups to strength training sessions, we exert a greater than normal *resistance* on them. When we lift heavy things, the stress exerted on our muscles causes muscle fibers to partially "break down" while our bodies release hormones that cause an inflammatory response. As a result of strength training, we may feel a "burn" or soreness in the affected muscles. A post-workout cool down with self-myofascial release (foam rolling) and static stretching will help to lessen muscle soreness.

By incorporating *rest* periods in between exercise sessions, we maximize the *recovery* process. During this 48-hour period, the body *repairs* the broken-down muscle fibers, aiding in muscle growth and strength. The repair period builds muscular strength through a repetitive cycle of resistance, rest, and recovery. Therefore, if you do strength training on major muscle groups (i.e. chest, back, legs), give them 48 hours of rest to allow them to recover and repair before repeating strength training on the same muscle groups. We will further discuss rest, recovery, and self-myofascial release in *Pillar 2: Recovery and Rest.*

STRENGTH-TRAINING TOOLS AND EQUIPMENT

Strength training can be accomplished through various tools and equipment. In the past, firefighters typically resorted to using weight machines and free weights. However, a functionally fit firefighter uses a wide array of strength training modalities:

> ▸ Firefighting equipment (SCBA harness/cylinder, fire hose, hand tools, hydraulic tools, saws, rope, ladders, etc.)
> ▸ Free weights (dumbbells, barbells, kettlebells)
> ▸ Bodyweight exercises (push-ups, pull-ups, core exercises, air squats, lunges, etc.)
> ▸ Weight machines or cable machines (preferred over weight machines)
> ▸ Resistance bands
> ▸ Medicine balls
> ▸ Suspension strap systems (TRX® or WOSS® straps)

COMPOUND VS. ISOLATION MOVEMENTS

A *compound movement* involves multiple muscle groups and joints. Compound movements are functional movements that help us to improve coordination, balance, and typically emphasize a total-body workout. Examples include squats, deadlifts, core and yoga exercises, and firefighting movements involving pushes, pulls, lifts, carries, and drags.

Let's examine the *squat* and explain why it is an ideal compound movement. When properly executing a squat, we involve our core, glutes (buttocks), quadriceps, hamstrings, and calf muscles. All of these muscles work together to successfully and safely complete the functional movement of lifting a heavy object off of the ground.

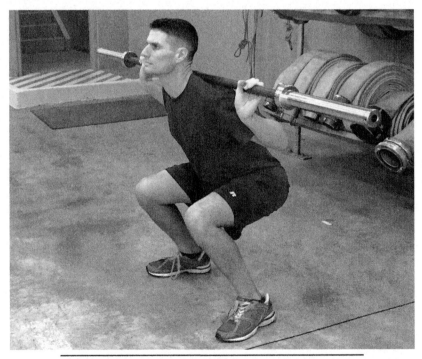

Compound Movements: The squat exercise uses multiple areas of the body for improvements in functional strength and performance.

An *isolation* movement only involves a single muscle and joint. These are movements that are typically performed on strength training machines in gyms. Bicep curls, leg extension, and hamstring (leg) curls are examples of isolation movements. These exercises may be ideal for bodybuilders, but they are not the best choices for a firefighter's functional fitness.

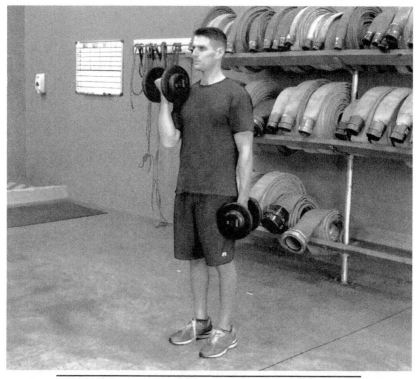

Isolation Movements: Bicep curls will increase muscular strength, but they are not the best choice for improving functional strength.

To make our fitness more functional, we want to focus on real-life, firefighter-specific movements. Very rarely do we use a single, isolated muscle when operating on the fireground. Instead, we use a combination of muscles and joints to accomplish the tasks at-hand. Therefore, functionally fit firefighters primarily focus on compound movements for building functional strength.

PROGRESSION AND REGRESSION METHODS

Functionally fit firefighters use progression and regression methods when completing strength training sessions. Nearly every functional strength training exercise can be *progressed* (made more difficult) or *regressed* (made less difficult) to suit individual fitness levels and goals. Doing so will maximize the benefit of the exercise by incrementally increasing its difficultly. Consider the following example of various ways to progress the *standing overhead press* exercise.

Assume a beginning weight of 20-pound dumbbells or kettlebells.

1. **Progressions**:
   A. Increase weight in 5-pound increments per set.
   B. Alternate arms when pressing overhead (i.e. right, left, right, left).
   C. Execute single-arm overhead press (i.e. right, right, right, right, left, left, left, left).
   D. Squat then overhead press.
   E. Step up to platform then overhead press.
   F. Balance on one leg with overhead press.
2. **Regressions**:
   A. Use a single barbell of equivalent weight instead of two dumbbells.
   B. Decrease the weight of the dumbbells or kettlebells.
   C. Execute seated overhead shoulder press (stability ball or bench seat)

Another example of a functional strength progression is demonstrated with the basic push-up. A beginner may start by executing push-ups with knees touching the ground, then progress to a standard push-up (feet on the ground). For advanced progressions, add weight to the back, elevate the legs on a bench or platform, do slow tempo push-ups (count to five as you move down and again as you push back up), and move the hands closer to the body's midline.

Whatever exercise we choose to execute, functionally fit firefighters understand the significance of using progressions and regressions. Doing so adds variety to our workouts and keeps our strength training interesting and dynamic.

8 TIPS FOR IMPROVING FUNCTIONAL STRENGTH

1. **Start small and build up slowly to avoid injury**. Listen to your body. If something hurts while you are executing a movement, stop immediately.

2. **Remember: Functional strength centers around the concept of *performance*, not building muscle**. Therefore, firefighters must separate themselves from the mindset of working out muscle groups (i.e. chest, arms, legs, etc.). Instead, we will focus on executing five fundamental firefighting movements during strength training: *pushing, pulling, lifting, carrying*, and *dragging*.

3. ***Proper form* leads to *proper function***. Correct form is always more important than using an excessive amount of weight. If the amount of weight causes your form to suffer, you are lifting too much weight, which can cause injuries.

4. **Focus on compound movements rather than isolation movements.** Most firefighting tasks and movements are centered on compound movements.

5. **Use multiple planes of motion for the same exercise**. For an upper-body pushing movement, push horizontally, vertically (both up and down), at an incline, and a decline. Using various directions of movement builds the dynamic strength functionally fit firefighters need.

6. **Strength training should be performed 3 to 5 times per week**. This can translate to one upper-body session, one lower-body session, and one total-body session per week. Do not perform strength training on the same major muscle group more than twice in one week.

7. **When possible, ensure 48 hours of rest before repeating strength training on the same muscle groups.** Remember: Rest, recovery, and repair are extremely important to improving our functional strength.

8. **When possible, perform movements that involve multiple muscle groups.** For example, do push-ups or standing cable chest press instead of supine bench press. The former exercises involve accessory muscles in the core and legs, which will improve balance and stability.

Functionally fit firefighters know strength training is undoubtedly one of the foundations of their physical fitness. Now that we have laid the foundation for building functional strength, we will continue our discussion of The Big 8 with The Push, Pull, Lift, Carry, and Drag.

ACTION STEPS:

1. Know the 4 R's of strength training and apply them to your functional strength training routines: resistance, rest, recovery, and repair

2. Understand the difference between compound and isolation movements and which are most important to firefighter functional fitness.

3. Commit to functional strength training sessions at least three times a week (e.g. upper-body, lower-body, total-body).

4. Utilize progression and regression methods to maximize your functional strength training sessions.

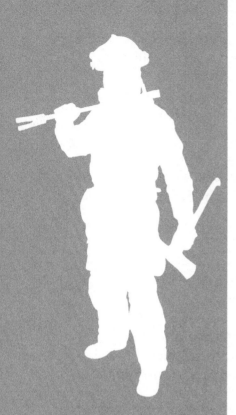

Want to be able to "make the push" on the fireground?

Then you must first "push" yourself in training.

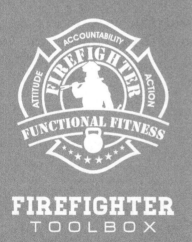

FIREFIGHTER
TOOLBOX

CHAPTER 8

THE BIG 8: THE PUSH

WHAT IS *THE PUSH*?

Pushing is one of the most fundamental movements for firefighters to execute. In layman's terms, a push is the act of exerting force on something to move it away from you or its starting location. A firefighter's pushing capacity, especially when mobility is restricted and environmental conditions are arduous, must *not* be taken for granted.

WHY IS *THE PUSH* IMPORTANT?

The Push is a critical movement for fireground tasks, both as a stand-alone movement and in combination with other movements. Functionally fit firefighters know the importance of strength training that directly applies to the many "push" movements required on the fireground.

COMMON FIREGROUND PUSH MOVEMENTS

> Ladder raises
> Hose line handling and advancement
> Forcible entry (striking, defeating doors, etc.)
> Ventilation (chopping or striking roofs and windows)
> Overhaul of ceilings and walls
> Self-rescue techniques

When pushing, we rely on the following areas and muscles of our bodies:

> Upper arm (triceps brachii)
> Chest (pectoralis major and minor)
> Shoulder (deltoid)
> Core
> Legs (biceps femoris, rectus femoris, gluteus maximus, gastrocnemius)

HOW TO INCREASE PUSH STRENGTH

We improve our push capacity by focusing on functional strength training exercises that build muscular strength, endurance, and power specifically for pushing movements. In other words, we use pushing exercises that mimic fireground tasks as opposed to those that build "beach bodies." If you want to be functionally fit, increase your push capacity by incorporating the exercises listed below into your strength training routines.

TOP 10 EXERCISES
TO IMPROVE FUNCTIONAL PUSH STRENGTH

1) Push-ups

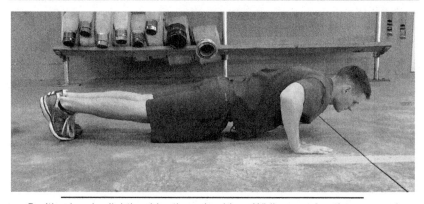

Position hands slightly wider than shoulders. While engaging the core and maintaining a neutral spine, lower the chest to a fist's distance above the ground.

- **Progressions**: Feet elevated, weight on back, hands wide, hands together, hands up at ear level, yoga (chaturanga) push-ups, slow tempo push-ups, Bosu® or stability ball push-ups, push-ups with suspension straps
- **Regressions**: Knees and feet on ground, standing chest press with cable machine (with light weight)

2) Dips

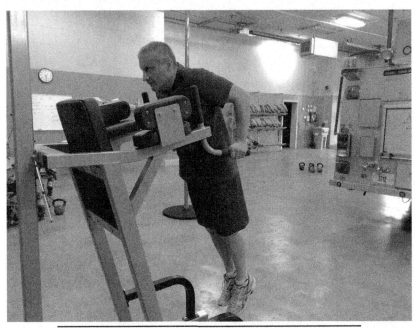

Lower the body until the elbows bend at 90 degrees.

- **Progression**: Weighted dips, slow tempo dips
- **Regressions**: "Assisted" dip with resistance bands under feet or with dip-assist machine

3) Standing Overhead Press

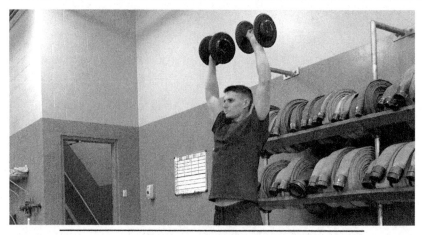

While engaging the core, push dumbbells, barbell, or kettlebells straight overhead.

> **Progressions**: Alternate arms, single-arm, kettlebell push-press, balance on single leg, squat then overhead press

> **Regressions**: Seated overhead press on bench or on stability ball, use single barbell, shoulder press weight machine

4) Ladder Raise and Lower

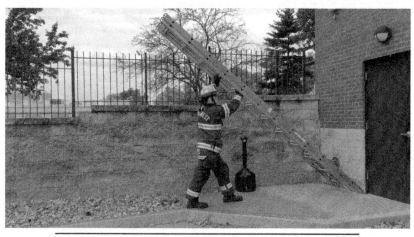

Place butt of ladder against building. Going rung by rung, raise the ladder until it is vertical. Reverse the process to lower the ladder to the ground.

> **Progression**: Add and secure weight to top of ladder, squat while holding ladder at chest-level and then raise it

> **Regression**: Choose a lighter ladder (e.g. roof or attic)

5) Medicine Ball Squat Press and Throw

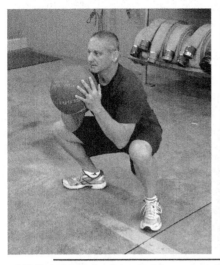 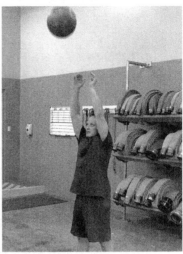

While holding medicine ball in center of chest, lower the body into a squat position. Explode upwards and simultaneously throw the medicine ball overhead. Let the medicine ball fall to the ground.

> **Progressions**: Use heavier medicine ball
> **Regressions**: Use lighter medicine ball, medicine ball throw without a squat

6) Squats

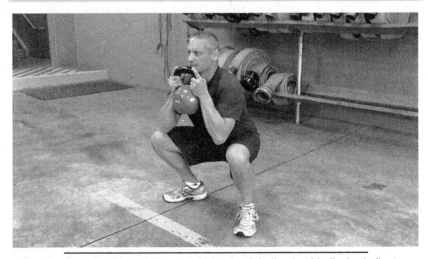

Position feet shoulder-width apart. Using kettlebells, dumbbells, barbell, etc., squat down to chair height and then stand back up.

> **Progressions**: Single-leg squat (no weight), single-leg squat to touchdown (no weight), single-leg Romanian deadlift, increased weight, reps, and rounds, increase depth of the squat at the bottom
> **Regressions**: Air squats (no weight), reduce depth of squat, squats with arms holding suspension straps for balance

7) Step-ups

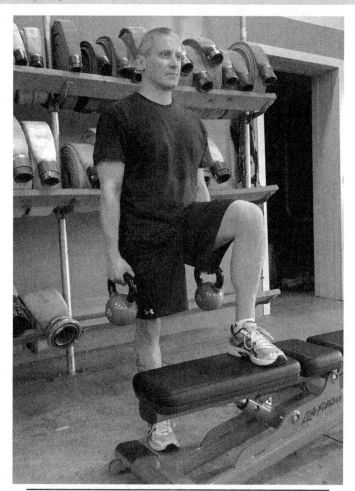

Using a bench, box or pedestal, step up and down.

> **Progressions**: Holding weight in both arms, holding weight in one arm, holding weight overhead, step-up to balance on one leg, increase step height
> **Regressions**: Lower height of step, ascend standard stairs

8) Sledgehammer Strike

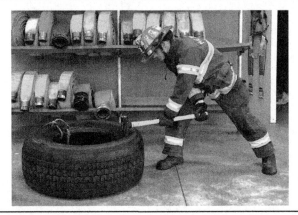

Forcefully strike a rubber tire with both arms leading. Can be performed in a standing (overhead) position, standing (lateral) position, standing on top of tire striking downwards, and kneeling on the ground (forcible entry simulation).

> **Progressions**: Use heavier sledgehammer, kneeling strike, standing lateral (side) strike
> **Regression**: Use lighter sledgehammer or lighter striking tool

9) Lunges

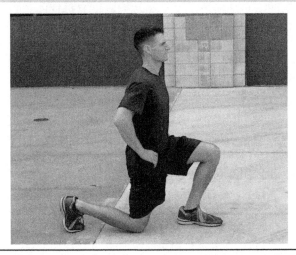

For a forward lunge (pictured), extend the front leg forward and dip the center of the body downward. At the lowest position, the front knee should not go past the tips of the toes.

> **Progressions**: Walking lunges, weighted lunges, using weight on only one side, weight held overhead, reverse

121

lunges, side lunges, balance on one leg when coming to standing position, overhead wood-chopper lunge with dumbbell

› **Regression**: Use step box or platform for front foot to reduce depth of lunge

10) Sled Push with Gym Mat

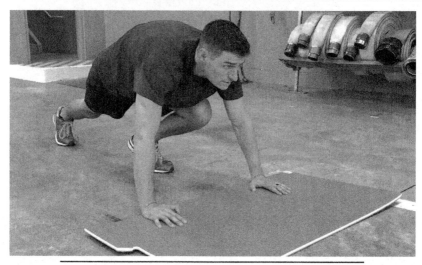

Use a gym mat that easily slides on a smooth floor. Extend the arms and push the mat, using the legs. Push the mat 25-100 feet in distance.

› **Progression**: Add weight to the mat, increase distance
› **Regression**: Shorten the distance

You may notice that pushing exercises such as the *bench press, tricep extension*, and *calf raises* are not included in the list above. There is very good reason for this: We want firefighters to use their core and legs for stability when pushing with their upper bodies. Performing exercises like the bench press do not adequately incorporate the core and legs.

When we are on the fireground, we do not execute pushing movements while lying flat on our back. So why should we perform pushing exercises while lying on a bench? As for the tricep extension, this exercise may help build upper-arm physique, but it is not very functional. If you are concerned about neglecting your triceps, know that every upper-body push exercise listed above uses the triceps as synergists (i.e. accessory muscles that help complete the movement). Lastly, calf raises are purely for improving physique, not function. Exercises such as step-ups, lunges, squats, deadlifts, and ascending stairs all build functional calf strength that firefighters *can actually use* on the fireground.

Pushing exercises, like all functional strength exercises, can be programmed in many ways. Functionally fit firefighters combine pushing and pulling exercises in alternating sets to focus on one area of the body (e.g. upper-body push/pull workout). Conversely, a total-body push workout incorporates both the upper body and lower body.

To program either an upper-body or lower-body push workout, choose 4 to 5 push exercises that apply. Perform 3 to 4 sets of each exercise for a total of 12 to 20 sets. The amount of repetitions for each exercise will vary, depending on the exercise being performed and its intensity or resistance. Get creative, have fun, and "push" yourself.

ACTION STEPS:

1. Use *The Push* exercises found in this section to increase functional push capacity.

2. Perform at least one upper-body push workout and one lower-body push workout per week. If you are feeling ambitious, combine both into the same session for a total-body push workout.

3. Give affected muscle groups 48 hours of rest to recover after your workouts before performing strength training on the same muscle groups.

4. Avoid strength training exercises that do not directly improve fireground function.

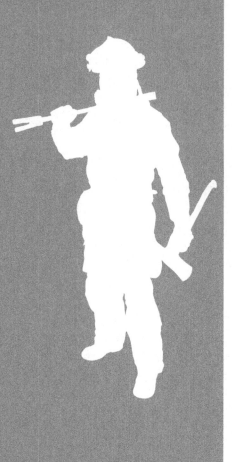

Functionally fit firefighters understand that pulling movements occur throughout an incident—from the initial hose line stretch through overhaul, mop-up, and even cleaning and restoring equipment back at the station.

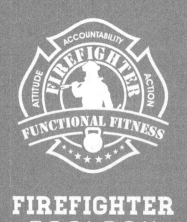

FIREFIGHTER
TOOLBOX

CHAPTER 9
THE BIG 8: THE PULL

WHAT IS *THE PULL*?

The Pull is another fundamental functional movement for firefighters. Simply speaking, a pull involves holding on to something and moving it in a particular direction, especially towards you. Firefighters execute pull movements frequently during firefighting operations. Like *The Push*, it is regularly combined with other movements, such as lifting, carrying, and dragging.

WHY IS *THE PULL* IMPORTANT?

Often, pulls are executed repeatedly and while firefighters are in awkward body positions—thus re-emphasizing the importance of a strong core for stability and injury prevention. Pulls are required throughout an incident; therefore, firefighters also need sufficient cardiovascular capacity to maintain work effectiveness and efficiency.

Functionally fit firefighters understand that pulling movements occur throughout an incident—from the initial hose line stretch through overhaul, mop-up, and even cleaning and restoring equipment back at the station. A firefighter's functional strength training must enhance pulling capacity.

COMMON FIREGROUND PULL MOVEMENTS

> Hose line pulling, handling, and advancement
> Overhaul of ceilings, walls, soffits, etc.
> Horizontal ventilation
> Prying objects
> Victim removal
> Self-rescue techniques
> Extension ladder raises
> Equipment and tool hoisting

Common muscle groups that are engaged with pulling exercises include:

> Upper arm (biceps brachii)
> Forearm and hands (digitorum profundus, digitorum superficialis, digiti minimi brevis, pollicis longus)
> Upper back (latissimus dorsi)
> Core
> Shoulder (deltoid and trapezius)
> Legs (biceps femoris, rectus femoris, gluteus maximus, gastrocnemius)

HOW TO INCREASE PULL STRENGTH

When training to improve pull strength, a primary consideration is to think about the positioning of our arms and how it affects our ability to execute the movement with proper force (e.g. overhead, cantilever position in front of body, left or right side dominant, etc.). Once again, body positioning also underscores the importance of core strength and stability.

Functionally fit firefighters will improve their pull capacity by focusing on strength training exercises that build muscular strength, endurance, and power specifically for pulling movements that are commonly required on the fireground. To continually improve your functional fitness, use pulling exercises that directly mimic fireground tasks, rather than using exercises that primarily build physique.

TOP 10 EXERCISES TO IMPROVE FUNCTIONAL PULL STRENGTH

1) Pull-ups

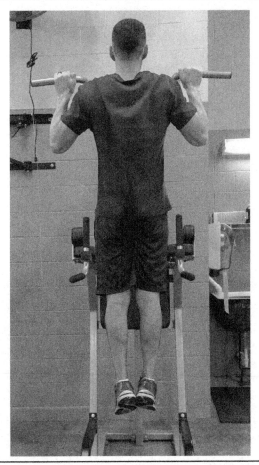

With palms facing away, grasp pull-up bar. While engaging the core, raise chin above bar. Avoid excessive swaying. If unable to complete a pull-up, use a pull-up assist machine or exercise bands to decrease the resistance.

> **Progressions**: Weighted with SCBA harness or vest, L-hang (legs extended forward), slow tempo pull-ups

> **Regressions**: Dead hangs, tension holds, pull-up assist devices (machine or elastic bands), kneeling or seated cable pull-downs

2) Equipment Hoist

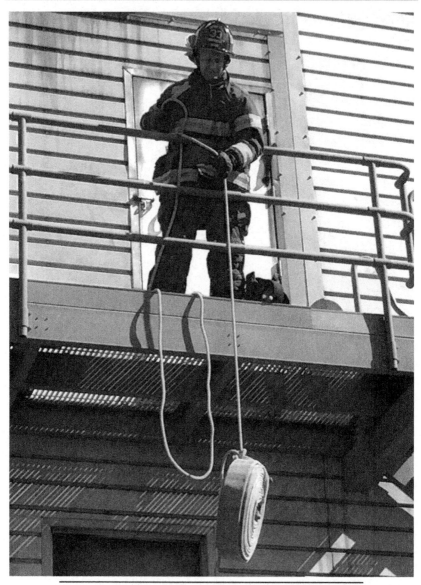

From an elevated walkway (with railing), hoist and lower equipment or hose with a rope. Alternatively, hoist and lower hose bundles with rope in your fire station's hose tower (if equipped with a pulley system).

> **Progressions**: Use heavier equipment or weight, wear firefighter PPE

> **Regressions**: Single-arm or alternating-arm cable pull-downs

3) Charged Attack Hose Pull

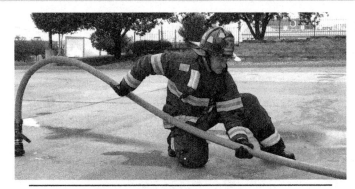

From a kneeling position, pull a charged attack hose (hand-over-hand). Reset the hose and switch sides.

> **Progressions**: Larger diameter attack hose, uncharged large diameter supply hose

> **Regressions**: Lighter attack hose, lightweight kneeling cable pull

4) Single-arm Angled Cable Row

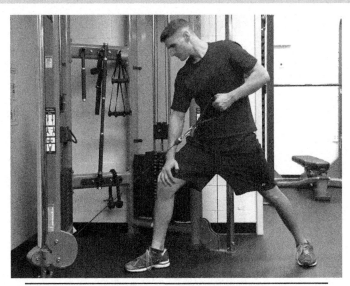

From a standing position, lean forward with your hips. Engage your core and pull the weight towards your side. This movement is intended to simulate starting a chainsaw or rotary saw. Perform movement on both sides.

> **Progressions**: Heavier weight, alternating arms

> **Regression**: Two-arm seated cable row

129

5) Double Kettlebell Swing

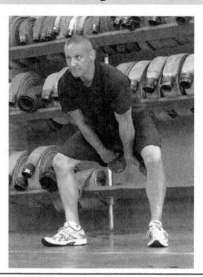

Grasp the kettlebells firmly. Engage your core and use the momentum of your hips as a hinge to thrust the kettlebells upward. Do not use your shoulders or arms to "lift" the kettlebells—the movement should come from the hips and core.

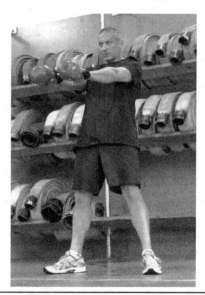

Completed movement.

> **Progression**: Heavier kettlebells, one-arm kettlebell swing
> **Regression**: Lighter kettlebells, two-hand single kettlebell swing

6) Deltoid/Reverse Fly

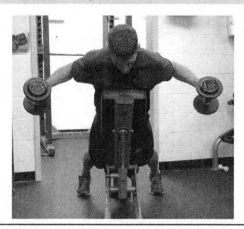

Putting the front of the torso against an angled bench,
lift dumbbells upward and outward.

> **Progression**: Bent-over standing fly
> **Regressions**: With suspension straps (TRX®), seated
  machine fly, arms only (no weight)

7) Battle Hose

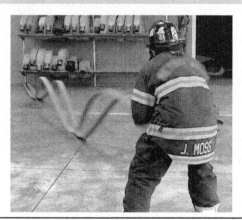

In a standing athletic position, whip a 50-foot section of attack hose
that is anchored at its midpoint. Quickly alternate hands in an up-down motion,
and use large sweeping movements. Perform the exercise for 15-60 seconds.

> **Progressions**: Larger diameter hose, longer hose, longer
  duration
> **Regressions**: Smaller and shorter hose, shorter duration

8) Kneeling Lateral Cable Pull

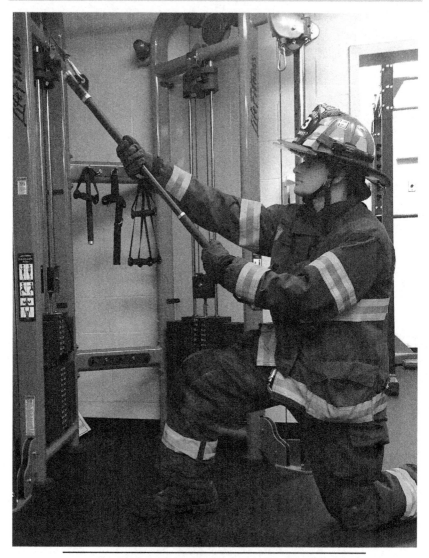

Use this movement to simulate pulling ceiling.
Perform the movement on both sides.

> **Progressions**: Standing position, change direction of pull (high/low)

> **Regressions**: Seated two-hand cable pull

9) Bent-Over Row

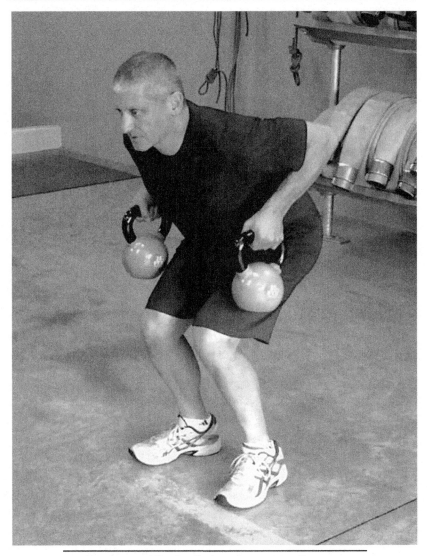

Bend over while simultaneously engaging the core.
Pull weights towards the sides of your torso.

> **Progressions**: Perform on BOSU® platform to challenge stability

> **Regressions**: Single-arm bent over rows, single-arm angled cable row, rowing machine, seated cable row

10) Inverted Rows

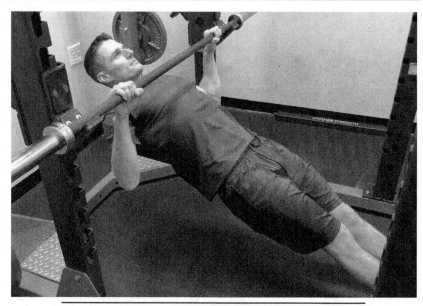

This is a horizontal version of a standing cable row. With a barbell secured to a squat rack, lower yourself all the way down so that your arms are fully extended. Pull your chest to touch the bar.

> **Progressions**: Position hands further apart (wide grip) position body more parallel (lower) to the ground, elevate feet on a platform or box, wear weighted vest or SCBA harness

> **Regressions**: Position body more perpendicular to the ground (standing and leaning back), use suspension straps (TRX®)

Pulling exercises, like all strength-training exercises, can be programmed in many ways. Push and pull exercises can be combined as alternating strength training sets to focus on one area of the body (e.g. upper-body push-pull strength workout). Alternatively, a total-body "pull workout" will use both the upper body and lower body, incorporating exercises listed above with additional lifting, carrying, and dragging exercises.

In order to provide variety and directly relate functional movements to firefighting tasks, use fireground tools and equipment to complement your workout sessions. An added benefit to exercising with firefighting tools is that it builds muscle memory and sharpens firefighting skills. With the equipment we have on-hand in the station, we can easily design exercises to improve our pulling capacity.

To program a pull workout, choose 4 to 5 pull exercises that apply to common fireground tasks. Perform 3 to 4 sets of each exercise for a total of 12 to 20 sets. The total amount of repetitions depends on the following acute variables: the specific exercise or movement, your current level of functional strength, your choice of progression, and the intensity of the exercise. You are only limited by your creativity. Pulling exercises can be completed with just about anything you can find in the fire station as well as with traditional exercise equipment. Be safe, do what you like, and keep it functional!

ACTION STEPS:

1. Survey your fire station and identify at least five opportunities to execute functional pulling exercises with the equipment you have on hand.

2. Use the pull exercises found in this section to increase your functional pull strength.

3. After your workouts, give the affected muscle groups 48 hours of rest to fully recover before using them again for the same type of strength training.

4. Remember to focus on core stability, balance, and posture while performing pull exercises to avoid injury to your back.

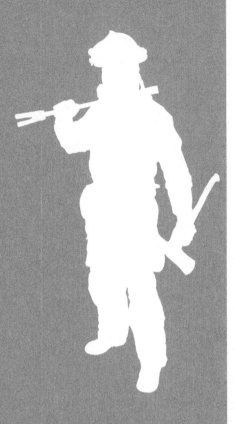

As a firefighter, you are at a greater risk of suffering a back injury.

Preparation and prevention are keys to protecting yourself from becoming one of these statistics.

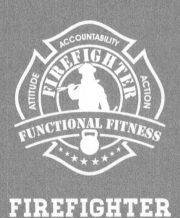

FIREFIGHTER
T O O L B O X

CHAPTER 10
THE BIG 8: THE LIFT

WHAT IS LIFTING?

Lifting generally refers to raising objects. Functionally fit firefighters apply this simple definition to common firefighting tasks and train to improve their ability to carry them out.

WHY IS LIFTING IMPORTANT?

The act of lifting has the greatest potential for injuring firefighters, especially when we are fatigued. We frequently lift people and heavy pieces of equipment, both on and off the fireground. Numerous studies point to back injuries (particularly strains and sprains), as the leading firefighter injury.

Proper Body Mechanics

The physical requirements of our profession are such that we cannot avoid lifting heavy objects, resulting in a high percentage of fire and EMS personnel who injure their back in the line of duty. It is vitally important for us to have proper body mechanics and strength so that we can successfully perform our duties, preserve our back, and thrive on the fireground throughout our careers.

Warning: When it comes to lifting, there is more to it than simply being strong enough to hoist an object. Unfortunately, lifts are often executed with awkward and non-ideal body positions when we are performing our duties.

Here are some statistics at a glance[6]:

> ➤ Back problems are among the most common and *most expensive* work-related injuries in the United States.
> ➤ Firefighters are at an increased risk of back injury as compared to other professions.
> ➤ Each year, approximately 50 percent of firefighter line-of-duty injuries are sprains and strains.
> ➤ *Annually, back injuries account for almost 50 percent of all firefighter line-of-duty retirements.*

As a firefighter, you are at a greater risk of suffering a back injury. Preparation and prevention are keys to protecting yourself from becoming one of these statistics.

COMMON FIREFIGHTER LIFTING MOVEMENTS

- ➤ Picking up charged hose lines
- ➤ Lifting and raising ladders
- ➤ Lifting power saws and forcible entry tools from ground level
- ➤ Removing vehicle extrication equipment from apparatus
- ➤ Lifting fire extinguishers and appliances
- ➤ Hoisting high-rise packs
- ➤ Lifting patients and rescuing victims
- ➤ Rescuing downed firefighters

HOW TO IMPROVE LIFTING CAPACITY

First and foremost, functionally fit firefighters use the following tips for safe-lifting practices.

10 Tips for Safe Lifting

1. Keep your back as straight as possible to maintain spinal integrity. Avoid "rounding" the back or "hunching over" the object.
2. Form a stable base with the feet apart (shoulder-width, if possible).

3. Get close to your object and lift with the legs, using the quadriceps and hamstrings.

4. Engage the core and glutes (buttocks).

5. Use help when you can. If someone can assist you, let them.

6. Use power-assisted equipment whenever practical.

7. Use ergonomic equipment, handles, and straps to assist you with lifting properly.

8. Pivot under heavy objects when appropriate (e.g. ground ladder shoulder carry).

9. Think about driving your heels into the ground instead of the balls of your feet. This enhances stability.

10. Create a solid foundation. Strengthen your core and legs through frequent strength training.

TOP 10 EXERCISES TO IMPROVE LIFT TECHNIQUE AND CAPACITY

Functionally fit firefighters engage in a variety of exercises that serve to improve their occupational lifting capacity and reduce the chances of injury caused by improper lifting techniques.

1) Deadlifts

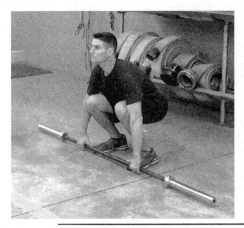 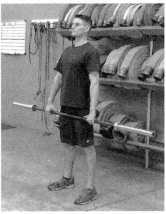

With a barbell, dumbbells or kettlebells on the floor, squat down and grab the weight. Engage the core and thrust your body upward, lifting the weight to a full standing position. Do not curve your back when lifting the weight.

- > **Progressions**: Increased weight, reps, and rounds, kettlebells in between the legs, kettlebells on the sides of the body
- > **Regressions**: Decreased weight, reps, and rounds, air squats

2) Dumbbell Scaptions

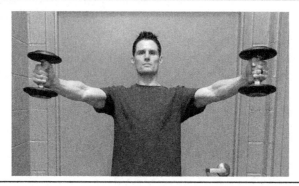

Stand with feet shoulder-width apart. Raise dumbbells in a Y-formation in front of the body until they are parallel to the ground. Arms should be straight.

- > **Progressions**: Balancing on a single-leg, alternating arms, single-arm scaptions, increased weight, reps, and rounds
- > **Regressions**: Seated position, decreased weight, reps, and rounds

3) Lunges

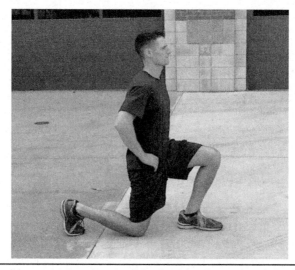

For a forward lunge (pictured), extend the front leg forward and dip the center of the body downward. At the lowest position, the front knee should not go past the tips of the toes.

> **Progressions**: Weighted, walking, reverse, side, lunge to balance on a single leg
> **Regressions**: Decreased weight, reps, and rounds

4) Hose Lifts for Shoulder Load Carries

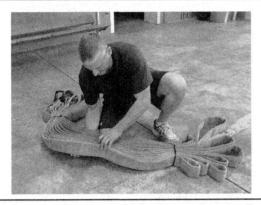

While squatting down and engaging the core, lift hose bundle off of ground. Place bundle on shoulder and stand up. Repeat on opposite side of body.

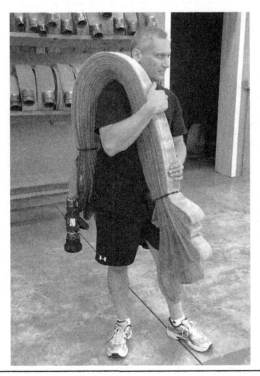

Completed movement.

› **Progressions**: Heavier hose, more rounds, lifting then carrying hose bundle on level ground and up elevations

› **Regressions**: Lighter hose, less reps, less rounds

5) Ladder Lift and Carry Variations

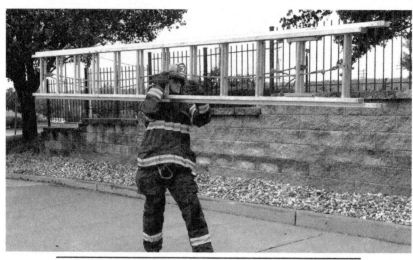

Over-the-Shoulder Ladder Lift: The ladder is lifted and balanced with the *outer* beam on top of the shoulder. Repeat on opposite side of body.

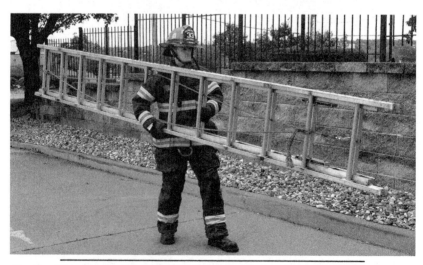

On-the-Shoulder Ladder Lift: The ladder is lifted and balanced with the *inner* beam on top of the shoulder. Repeat on opposite side of body.

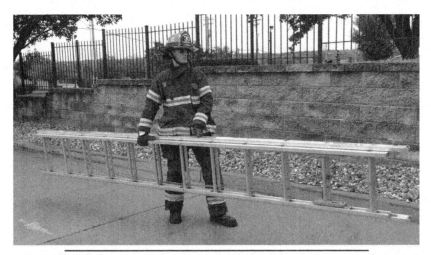

Ladder Lift and Carry on Side: The ladder is lifted and carried at the firefighter's side with the arms straight down. Repeat on opposite side of body.

> ➤ **Progressions**: Heavier ladders, more rounds, lift, carry, and ladder raise

> ➤ **Regressions**: Lighter ladders, less reps, less rounds

6) Heavy Tool Lifts and Carries

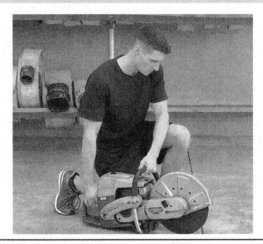

While squatting down and engaging the core, lift the tool off of the floor to a standing position. Repeat on opposite side of body.

➤ **Progressions**: Increased tool weight, two-tool lifts, increased reps, increased rounds

➤ **Regressions**: Lighter tools, single tool lifts, less reps, less rounds

7) Squats

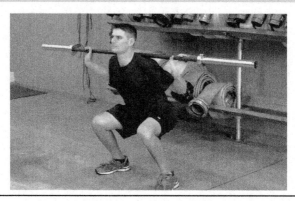

Position feet shoulder-width apart. Using kettlebells, dumbbells, barbell, etc., squat down to chair height and then stand back up.

> **Progressions**: Single-leg squat, single-leg squat to touchdown, single-leg Romanian deadlift, increased weight, reps, and rounds, increase depth of squat at the bottom

> **Regressions**: Air squats, prisoner squats, decreased weight, reps, and rounds

8) Upright Row

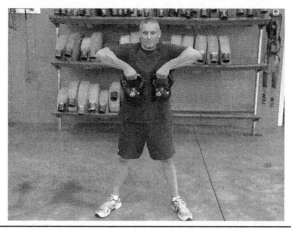

From a standing position, hold a barbell, dumbbells or kettlebells in front of the body at the hips. Pulling straight up, lift the weight to the chest.

> **Progressions**: Single-arm, alternating arms, balancing on single leg, increased weight, reps, and rounds

> **Regressions**: Decreased weight, reps, and rounds

9) Patient Lifts and Transfers

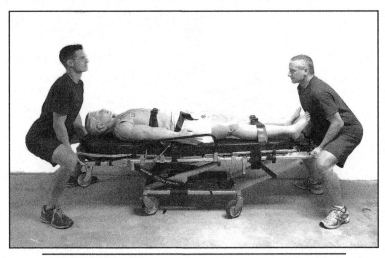

Using a partner, squat down to lift a stretcher with a weighted mannequin.

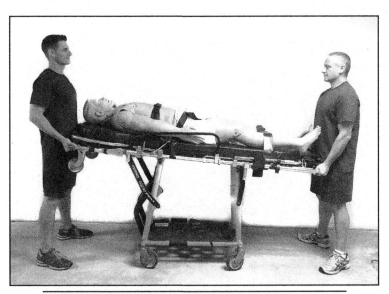

Completed movement.

> **Progressions**: Increased weight, more reps, varied heights, more rounds, lift and carry
> **Regressions**: Decreased weight, reps, and rounds

145

10) Plank Variations

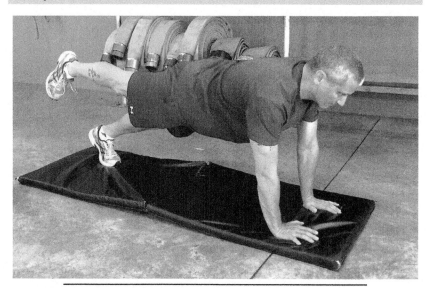

Three-Point Plank: Elevate single leg and hold. Maintain full-body tension.

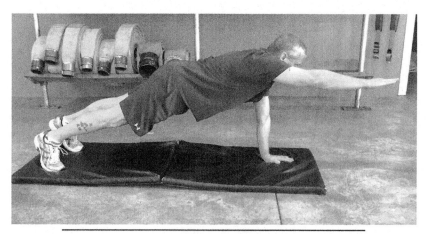

Three-Point Plank: Elevate single arm and hold. Maintain full-body tension.

> **Progressions**: Increased duration, side planks, three-point plank, two-point plank, plank on fingertips
> **Regressions**: Decreased duration, forearm planks, plank with knees on the ground

Functionally fit firefighters also know the purpose of practicing proper lifting techniques goes beyond the fireground. One of the objectives of firefighter functional fitness is to assist the firefighter in transitioning to a long and healthy retirement. The movements listed above, if practiced properly, will improve lifting technique. Eventually, this will develop muscle memory to the point where we should not have to consciously think about it before we execute a lift.

We must also practice lifts and proper lifting techniques while wearing our turnout gear and SCBA. We can accomplish this by lifting fireground tools and equipment. With the equipment we have on hand in the station, we can easily design exercises to improve our lifting capacity.

Finally, traditional strength training exercises that strengthen our core and legs will also improve our lifting capacity. Throughout our careers, proper lifting techniques will improve our fireground performance, and they will reduce our risk of chronic injuries that could negatively impact our lifestyles.

ACTION STEPS:

1. **Use the lifting exercises found in this section to increase your functional lifting capacity.**

2. **Memorize and adopt the 10 tips for safe lifting. Use them consistently.**

3. **Combine lifting exercises with your carry exercises to increase your cardiovascular capacity. Lift an object, and then carry it a specific distance on level ground or up/down an elevation, depending on your level of fitness.**

4. **Remember to focus on core stability, balance, and posture while performing lifting movements and exercises to avoid injury to your back.**

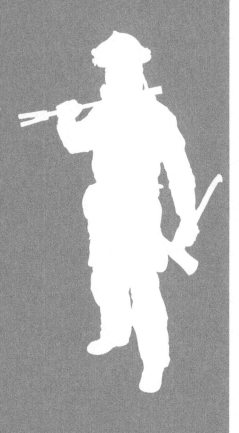

Wearing personal protective equipment reduces a firefighter's maximum physical performance by 25 percent and increases metabolic expenditure by 50 percent.

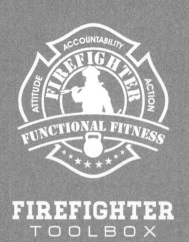

FIREFIGHTER
TOOLBOX

CHAPTER 11
THE BIG 8: THE CARRY

WHAT IS A CARRY?

As we continue our discussion of firefighter functional fitness, it is worth noting that many of the movements we have already discussed are ballistic in nature. In other words, we are required to use muscular strength and endurance to execute high-velocity, short duration movements in a repetitious manner.

In this section, we will shift gears as we focus on *The Carry*. While carries are not ballistic movements by definition, they are the most universal of all functional movements that relate to firefighting tasks, making them equally important in increasing overall functional fitness.

To carry is the task of holding something and moving with it. Functionally fit firefighters understand that our effective work capacity is greatly improved when we are able to efficiently carry heavy loads over a variety of elevations and terrains.

WHY IS CARRYING IMPORTANT FOR FIREFIGHTERS?

In the Swedish study *Firefighters' Physical Work Capacity*, Ann-Sofie Lindberg specifically identifies hose-carrying up flights of stairs and carrying equipment over terrain as two tests that aid in predicting a firefighter's overall work capacity. The study also points out that firefighters indicated these carrying tasks to be both highly difficult and extremely important to the job[7].

We teach rookie firefighters to always get off of the rig with a tool in-hand. This comes down to simply being prepared for what may lie ahead. So, think for a minute about all of the different things that firefighters carry. It is likely that your list will look something like the following list.

Table 11.1 – WHAT FIREFIGHTERS CARRY
Hose
Ladders
Personal tools
Power saws
Forcible entry tools
Stokes basket
Vehicle extrication equipment
Rope
Fire extinguishers
Water appliances
High-rise or standpipe packs
Medical bags
Heart monitors
Patients
Victims
Firefighters

However, before you carry anything listed above, there is someone else you must consider: *YOU!* Functionally fit firefighters know that we will always start by carrying our own weight. Firefighters also carry a standard protective ensemble that includes a set of turnout coat and pants, boots, helmet, SCBA cylinder and mask, flashlight, portable radio, and pocket tools.

A recent study has shown wearing personal protective equipment (PPE) reduces a firefighter's maximum physical performance by 25 percent and increases metabolic expenditure by 50 percent[8].

Carrying our standard protective ensembles emphasizes why functional strength and cardiovascular capacity are critical to our job. Let's take a closer look in the following sections.

HOW MUCH WEIGHT DO FIREFIGHTERS CARRY?

Over the past 50 years, there have been significant technological advancements in firefighting turnout gear: greater coverage, greater heat resistance,

> **"Firefighters routinely carry more than 100 pounds of extra weight while operating on the fireground."**

integrated harnesses, bailout systems, etc. Unfortunately, these safety improvements have caused our PPE's weight to increase substantially.

In an experiment, we decided to weigh a firefighter in their full protective ensemble, a set of irons, and a fire extinguisher ("water can"). We outfitted the firefighter exactly how they would be dressed at a working fire. Here are the results:

> Protective ensemble (turnout gear, bailout system, helmet, radio, gloves, flashlight, pocket tools, SCBA cylinder and mask): **70 pounds**
> Set of irons (axe and halligan): **25 pounds**
> Fire extinguisher ("water can"): **30 pounds**

In this scenario, the firefighter would be carrying 125 pounds *in addition* to their own body weight. This is an extra 125 pounds that the firefighter will carry to their assignment on the fireground. Once they actually arrive at their assignment, they are then required to really "go to work" by forcing a door, executing a search, helping advance a hose line, etc.

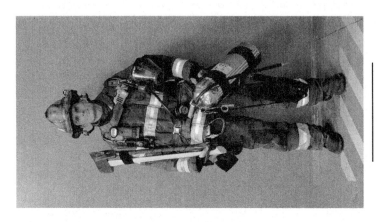

Firefighter with Irons and Water Extinguisher: The water extinguisher adds additional 30 pounds.

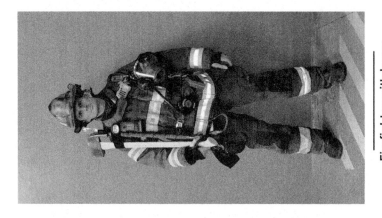

Firefighter with Irons: The axe and halligan add 25 pounds.

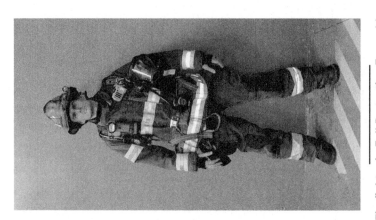

Firefighter in Full Protective Ensemble: Turnout gear, bailout system, helmet, radio, gloves, flashlight, pocket tools, SCBA cylinder and mask — 70 pounds.

THE ERGONOMICS OF CARRYING

Regardless of what you are carrying, one thing remains constant—we rarely carry anything in a symmetrical or balanced fashion. Even with the help of handles, straps, and other ergonomic devices designed to accommodate weight, our bodies will twist, shift, bounce, and adjust as we move. Depending on the equipment, we may execute carries at arm's length, at chest height, at shoulder height, above our head, or even a combination of positions at once. This serves as a reminder that optimal core strength is vitally important for executing all types of carries. A strong core will enhance our carrying power and reduce the risk of injury.

WHERE FIREFIGHTERS CARRY

From the fire station to fireground, carrying equipment is a fundamental aspect of the job. The obstacles we face when carrying things will challenge our strength, balance, mobility, flexibility, and cardiovascular capacity. The challenges we face while carrying our equipment include:

> Going up and down stairwells
> Ascending and descending ladders
> Traversing across, up, and down uneven or otherwise hazardous terrain
> Operating in constricted spaces
> Working under limited visibility
> Working in high-heat environments

Carries are required throughout an incident, requiring increased muscular and cardiovascular endurance. Terrain and environmental conditions also affect our ability to carry, often times making the simplest of tasks much more arduous while engaging multiple muscle groups at the same time.

Common muscle groups that are engaged with carries include:

> Legs (biceps femoris, rectus femoris, gluteus maximus, gastrocnemius)
> Core
> Upper back (latissimus dorsi)
> Upper arms (biceps brachii)
> Forearms and hands (digitorum profundus, digitorum superficialis, digiti minimi brevis, pollicis longus)
> Shoulders (deltoid and trapezius)

HOW TO IMPROVE FUNCTIONAL CARRYING CAPACITY

Functionally fit firefighters know that when training to improve carrying capacity they must carry things—*sometimes heavy things*. This includes carrying objects in offset positions, carrying asymmetrical loads, and combining our carries with changes of elevation as we increase our strength—these will improve muscle memory and increase balance.

In order to provide variety and directly relate functional movements to firefighting tasks, we carry fireground tools and equipment to complement our workout sessions. This can be done during skills training sessions and during specific fitness training sessions. Carrying firefighting tools and equipment builds muscle memory and sharpens our firefighting skills. With the equipment we have in the station, we can easily design exercises to improve our functional carrying capacity.

TOP 10 EXERCISES TO IMPROVE CARRYING CAPACITY

1) Farmer's Carry

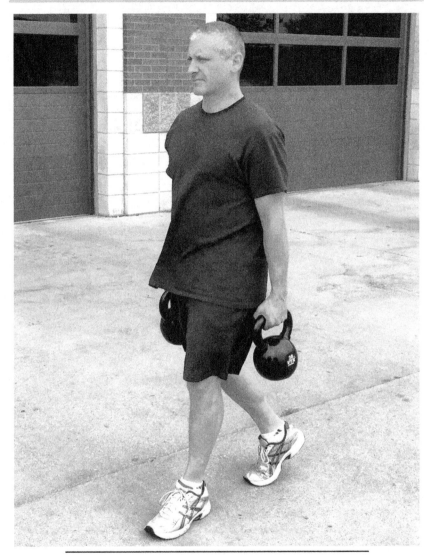

Carry dumbbells, kettlebells, or firefighting equipment
(i.e. saws, rescue tools) at arm's length.

> **Progressions**: Heavier weights, asymmetrical weights (heavier weight on one side of the body), carries wearing turnout gear and SCBA, elevation changes, increase distance
> **Regressions**: Lighter weights, decrease distance, level ground

155

2) Rack Hold Carry

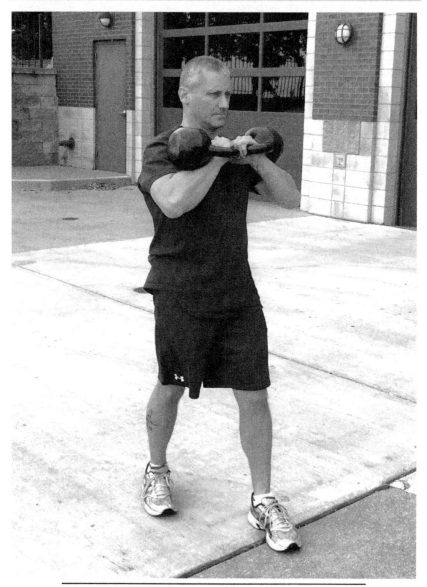

Carry kettlebells at chest height while engaging the core.

> **Progressions**: Heavier weights, asymmetrical weights, carries wearing turnout gear and SCBA, elevation changes, increase distance

> **Regressions**: Lighter weights, decrease distance, level ground

3) Overhead Carry

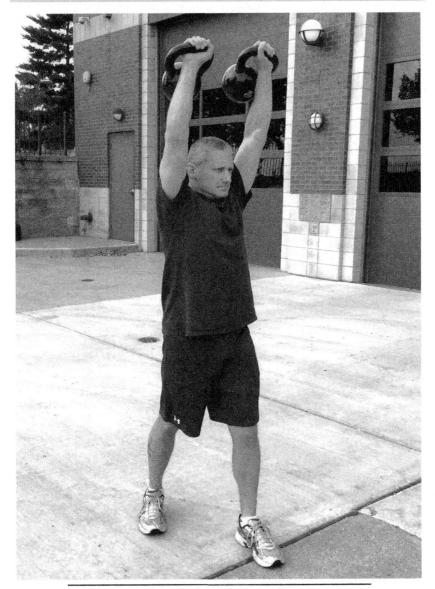

Carry weights with arms straight above your head. Engage the core.

> **Progressions**: Heavier weights, asymmetrical weights, single-arm carry, carries wearing turnout gear and SCBA, elevation changes, increase distance

> **Regressions**: Lighter weights, decrease distance, level ground

4) Shoulder Carry (100 foot of 1 3/4-inch hose)

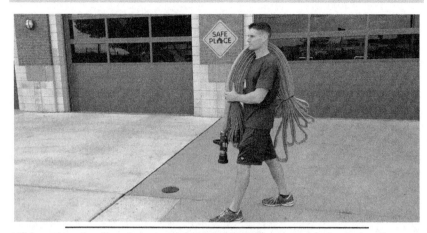

Lift hose bundle off and place on shoulder. Walk forward while engaging the core. Repeat movement on opposite shoulder.

> **Progressions**: Elevation changes (stairs), wearing turnout gear and SCBA, 2 1/2-inch hose bundle, increase distance

> **Regressions**: Level ground, decrease distance

5) Over-the-Shoulder Carry (ladder)

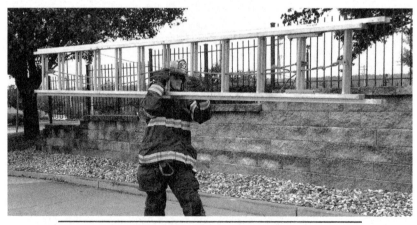

The ladder is lifted, balanced, and carried with the *outer* beam on top of the shoulder. Repeat on opposite side of body.

> **Progressions**: Elevation changes, wearing turnout gear and SCBA, heavier ladder, increase distance

> **Regressions**: Level ground, decrease distance, lighter ladder

6) On-the-Shoulder Carry (ladder)

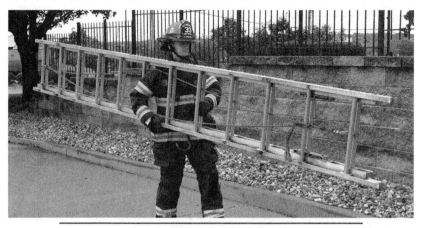

The ladder is lifted, balanced, and carried with the *inner* beam on top of the shoulder. Repeat on opposite side of body.

> **Progressions**: Elevation changes, wearing turnout gear and SCBA, heavier ladder, increase distance

> **Regressions**: Level ground, decrease distance, lighter ladder

7) Arm's-length Carry (ladder)

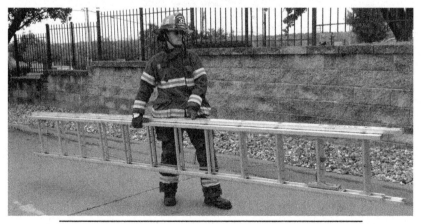

The ladder is lifted and carried at the firefighter's side with the arms straight down. Repeat on opposite side of body.

> **Progressions**: Elevation changes, wearing turnout gear and SCBA, heavier ladder, increase distance

> **Regressions**: Level ground, decrease distance, lighter ladder

8) Heavy Tool Carry

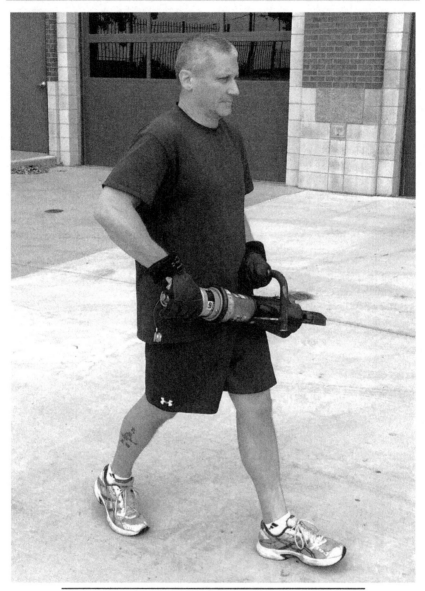

Carry heavy tool with both arms in front of body.

> **Progressions**: Heavier equipment, asymmetrical loads, carries wearing turnout gear and SCBA, elevation changes, increase distance

> **Regressions**: Lighter equipment, decrease distance, level ground

9) Weighted Lunges

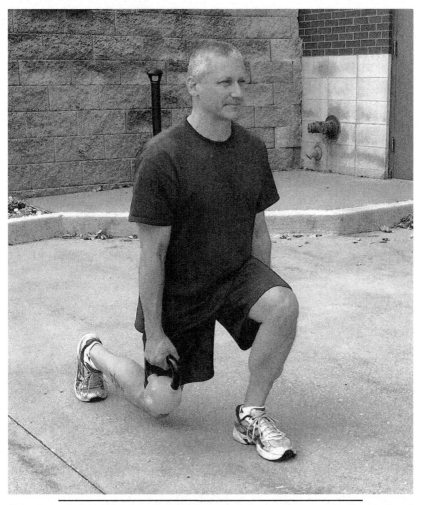

For a forward lunge (pictured), extend the front leg forward and dip the center of the body downward. At the lowest position, the front knee should not go past the tips of the toes.

> **Progressions**: Heavier weights, asymmetrical weights, carries wearing turnout gear and SCBA, elevation changes, increase distance or reps

> **Regressions**: Lighter weights, decrease distance or reps, level ground

10) Hose Carry on SCBA Cylinder

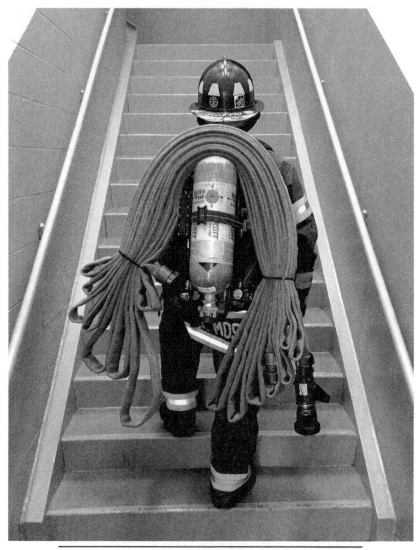

While wearing a SCBA cylinder, place hose bundle on top of cylinder.
Engage the core.

> **Progressions**: Elevation changes (stairs), wearing turnout
> gear in addition to SCBA, 2 1/2-inch hose bundle, increase
> distance

> **Regressions**: Smaller diameter hose, level ground,
> decrease distance

Carry exercises involve walking, but you can also carry objects a certain distance in one direction and drag an object back, crawl back, sprint back, or push something back to the starting point. These movements help to increase cardiovascular capacity and functional strength at the same time. Exercises to improve carrying capacity can be combined with sessions that also include cardiovascular capacity training, strength training, or any other functional movement practice.

ACTION STEPS:

1. Use *The Carry* exercises found in this chapter to increase your functional carrying capacity.

2. Combine carrying exercises with lifting, crawling, pushing, pulling, dragging, and sprinting exercises (e.g. carry in one direction, push, pull, drag, crawl, or sprint in the other direction) to increase your cardiovascular capacity.

3. Vary your carry weights and tool positions (arms-length, chest level, overhead, etc.) to mimic fireground functions. Always make sure you are safely executing carries from the best ergonomic position possible. Doing so will result in less fatigue.

4. Remember to build up core strength for stability, balance, and posture. These will help you execute carrying movements and prevent injury to your back.

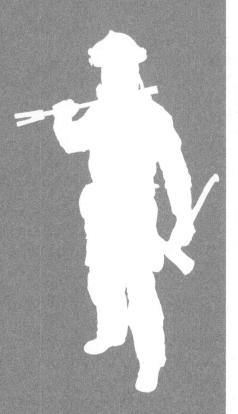

Functionally fit firefighters work smarter, not harder.

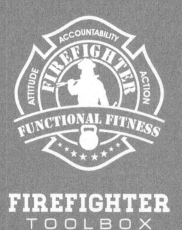

FIREFIGHTER
TOOLBOX

CHAPTER 12

THE BIG 8: THE DRAG

WHAT IS *THE DRAG?*

The drag is the act of moving something along a surface that simultaneously involves effort or pressure. As it pertains to firefighting duties that require dragging objects, we tend to think of activities that involve moving other people. Whether it is a victim, firefighter or piece of equipment, we cannot overstate the importance of having the muscular strength and endurance, flexibility, and cardiovascular capacity to execute these movements.

Although *The Drag* is probably one of the lesser used functional movements on the fireground, it is one of the *most important* to be able to execute properly and effectively. It can truly mean the difference between life and death. Functionally fit firefighters know that it is not only a *functional movement* but it is also a *life-saving skill.*

As with most functional movements, it is usually associated with companion movements. Specifically, dragging will most often be combined with lifting and carrying, and many of the exercises we discussed in previous sections will also apply to improving dragging capacity. However, like most things we want to improve upon, in order to become more efficient and effective with dragging, we must *actually drag* objects.

WHY IS DRAGGING CAPACITY IMPORTANT FOR FIREFIGHTERS?

Physical and Mental Impacts of the Drag

In the chapter on *The Lift,* we pointed out that sprains, strains, and back injuries were the primary causes for on-duty firefighter injuries and line-of-duty retirements. As such, we must always keep in mind that proper lifting techniques should also be used whenever possible as we prepare to drag equipment or people.

The increased cardiovascular capacity required while operating in restrictive equipment and difficult environments also limits us. The results of the study *The Influence of Self-Contained Breathing Apparatus on Ventilatory Function and Maximal Exercise* conclude that wearing and breathing from a SCBA restricts a firefighter's respiratory capacity—so much so that it will reduce aerobic performance by 15 percent[9].

" Wearing and breathing from an SCBA reduces aerobic performance by 15 percent."

The act of dragging a downed firefighter or victim will be among the most physically *and* mentally exhausting movements a firefighter will ever encounter. All of the stressors associated with these drags combine to impact our ability to effectively execute the task.

COMMON FIREFIGHTER DRAG MOVEMENTS

> Victim drag
> Firefighter drag
> Attack line drag (charged and uncharged)
> Supply line drag
> Ground ladder drag
> Rope drag
> Rapid Intervention Crew (RIC) pack drag

HOW TO IMPROVE DRAG CAPACITY

First and foremost, functionally fit firefighters work smarter, not harder. When it comes to dragging objects and people, being strong is only part of the equation. No matter the situation, dragging objects and people will drain your strength quickly, so here are some tips to help maximize your drag capacity and effectiveness.

8 Tips for Safe and Effective Dragging

1. Use additional manpower to assist (when possible).
2. Use the power of your legs to generate momentum.
3. Avoid or limit stopping once you have started moving.
4. Engage your core and maintain spinal integrity.
5. Lean into the object to take advantage of your body weight when dragging something forward, such as a charged hose line.
6. Use ergonomic equipment, handles, and straps to assist you (when possible).
7. Use as much leverage as possible. Avoid using the hand grip as your primary muscle group.
8. Avoid "rounding" your back or "hunching over" the object.

TOP 10 EXERCISES TO IMPROVE DRAG TECHNIQUE AND CAPACITY

1) Charged Attack Line Drag – Walking

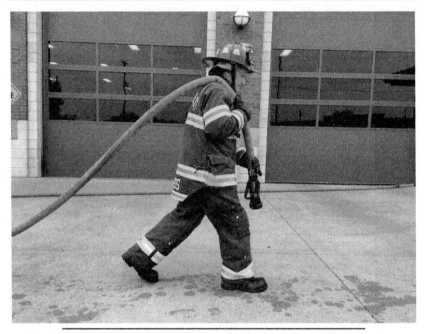

With a charged attack line over the shoulder,
lean forward and use your weight to create momentum.

› **Progressions**: Larger attack line (2 1/2-inch), increase distance, add elevation changes, operate hose line after dragging it

› **Regressions**: Smaller attack line (booster/forestry hose), decrease distance, level surfaces

2) Charged Attack Line Drag – Kneeling

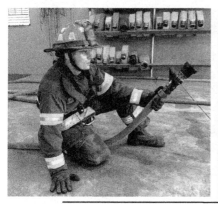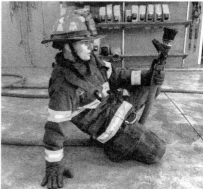

Left: While holding the nozzle in your left hand, place the hose under your right knee. Plant your right hand and left foot on the ground and advance the hose line by dragging your right leg forward.

Right: Using the right leg to drag the hose line forward.

> **Progressions**: Larger attack line (2 1/2-inch), increase distance, operate hose line after dragging it

> **Regressions**: Decrease distance

3) Charged Attack Line – Drag Up Stairs

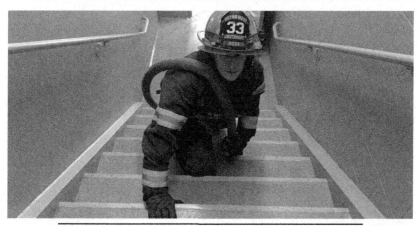

Loop the hose line over your shoulder and crawl and drag it up the stairs.

> **Progressions**: More flights of stairs, larger attack line, changes of direction, pull and push hose up stairs from a stationary position

> **Regressions**: Less flights of stairs, smaller attack line, uncharged hose line

169

4) Supply Line Drag

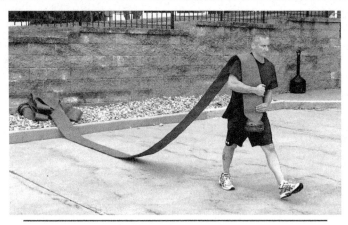

With the dry supply line over the shoulder,
lean forward and use your weight to create momentum.

> **Progressions**: Use 5-inch supply hose, longer hose line or drag distance

> **Regressions**: Use 3-inch supply hose, shorter hose line or shorter drag distance

5) Downed Firefighter Drag

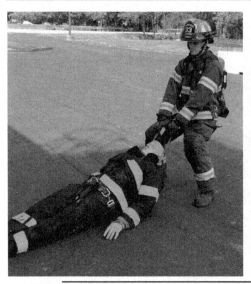 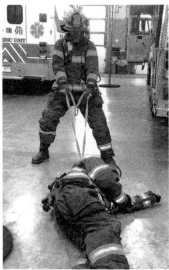

Left: Grab the downed firefighter's SCBA harness and drag backwards.
Right: Variation with webbing attached to downed firefighter's SCBA harness.

> **Progressions**: Crawl forward and drag firefighter with webbing, elevation changes, obstacles, obscured visibility, heavier weight, drag on a surface with greater friction

> **Regressions**: Drag firefighter on ground with webbing (walking backwards), level surface, shorter drag distance, lighter weight, drag on a surface with less friction

6) Victim Drag

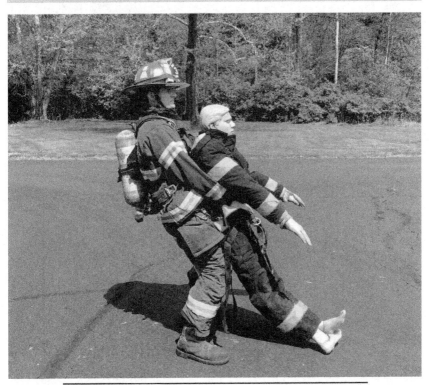

Pick victim up by the shoulders and drag backwards.

> **Progressions**: Hoist and drag victim from chest high position (walking backwards), elevation changes, obstacles, obscured visibility, heavier weight

> **Regressions**: Drag victim on ground with drag strap or webbing (walking backwards), level surface, shorter drag distance, lighter weight

7) Tire Drag

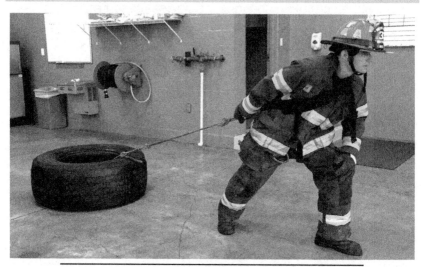

Forward Tire Drag: With a rope tied to a tire, lean forward and use your momentum to drag the tire.

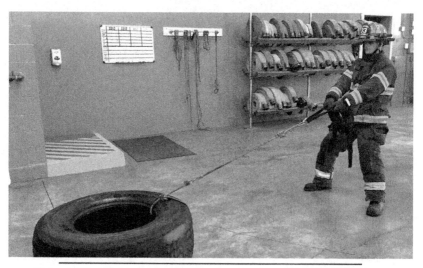

Reverse Tire Drag: Facing the tire, lean backwards and drag the tire.

> **Progressions**: Forward-facing drag, heavier tire, longer drag distance, more rounds

> **Regressions**: Rear-facing drag (walking backwards), lighter tire, shorter distance, less rounds

8) Deadlifts (barbell, kettlebell, dumbell)

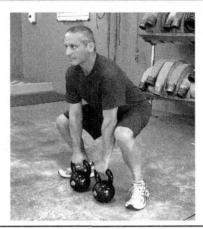

With a barbell, dumbbells or kettlebells on the floor, squat down and grab the weight. Engage the core and thrust your body upward, lifting the weight to a full standing position. Do not curve your back when lifting the weight.

> **Progressions**: Increase weight, reps, rounds

> **Regressions**: Decrease weight, reps, rounds

9) Standing Cable Row

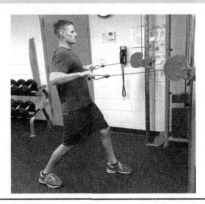

With a straight bar connected to a cable weight machine, pull resistance towards your body. Plant both feet firmly and engage your core.

> **Progressions**: Perform while on balancing on single leg, alternating arms, single-arm, increase weight and tension, reps, rounds

> **Regressions**: Seated cable row, rows with suspension straps (TRX®), decrease weight and tension, reps, rounds

10) Bear Crawl and Drag

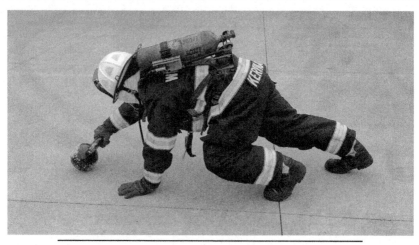

This is a combination of crawling like a bear and dragging a weight (i.e. kettlebell).

> **Progressions**: Increase distance, heavier drag object, wearing full turnout gear and SCBA

> **Regressions**: Decrease distance, lighter drag object

Performing drags on level surfaces and on changes in elevation are equally important skills that can be accomplished easily at a fire station and training facility. Remember, drags are a skill-based functional movement. Turnout gear and other equipment will realistically restrict our movements and challenge both our flexibility and cardiovascular capacity. Dragging a rescue dummy in gym clothing, for example, will provide a limited level of benefit. However, doing so while wearing our firefighting PPE will provide the most realistic conditions possible. For this reason, when practicing firefighter drag movements, functionally fit firefighters also execute drags while wearing their turnout gear and SCBA from time to time.

ACTION STEPS:

1. Use the 8 tips for safe and effective drags.

2. Use the dragging exercises found in this section to increase your functional drag capacity.

3. Use a variety of standard exercise equipment *and* firefighting tools and equipment when practicing drags.

4. Combine dragging exercises with lifting, crawling, pushing, pulling, and sprinting exercises to increase your cardiovascular capacity (drag an object a specific distance on level ground then crawl, push, pull, carry or sprint back).

5. Practice dragging rescue mannequins, people, and equipment while wearing turnout gear and breathing from an SCBA from time to time, once your level of fitness permits.

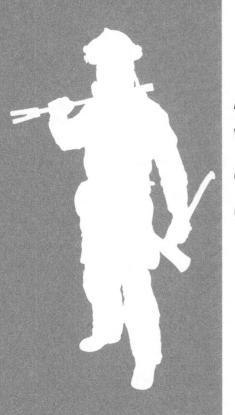

A one-hour workout is only 4 percent of your day.

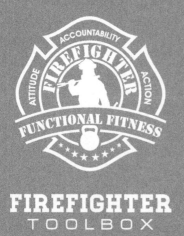

FIREFIGHTER
TOOLBOX

CHAPTER 13

PILLAR 2: RECOVERY AND REST

It is no secret that most firefighters dedicate the majority of their fitness training efforts toward *Pillar 1: Physical Fitness.* There are many good reasons for this. But, as much as we emphasize the physical aspects of our functional fitness training, we must also discuss the importance of the recovery process. Consider this: A one-hour workout is only 4 percent of the day. What we do with the other 96 percent of our time is equally, if not *more* important. How well we recover from our workouts plays a vital role in optimizing our functional fitness.

In this chapter, we will explain how to best utilize time *away* from the gym by incorporating passive and active recovery methods into daily routines. Passive recovery methods are those that do not require physical effort. On the other hand, active recovery methods may require physical exertion and specific actions to improve the recovery process.

WHAT IS PASSIVE RECOVERY?

Passive recovery methods are those that do not require any physical exertion on our part. The two primary avenues for passive recovery are *rest* and *sleep*. As firefighters, we are always on the go, and we seldom give our bodies and minds the opportunity to recharge. The same can be said for our weekly workouts. Although some may think that working out every day brings the most benefit, functionally fit firefighters know that rest days are an integral part of their fitness success.

We have good news: *Not only are rest and sleep important aspects of the recovery process but they are also the easiest to implement.*

WHY IS REST IMPORTANT FOR FIREFIGHTERS?

As discussed in the functional strength section, strength training causes microtears in our muscle fibers. Depending on the intensity of exercise performed and your current level of fitness, the body's natural inflammation process may also cause muscle soreness. Functionally fit firefighters understand that performing intense strength training on the same muscles too soon does not allow adequate time for rebuilding, repair, and recovery. Overtraining muscles and joints is a very real concern. It will lead to injury and serious setbacks if we do not incorporate adequate rest.

HOW TO INCORPORATE EFFECTIVE REST INTO YOUR ROUTINES

Functionally fit firefighters use the two following concepts to get the most recovery out of their rest:

Rest in between strength training sessions:

For strength training, strive for 48 hours of rest for affected muscle groups in between sessions. For example, if you perform upper-body "push" strength training on a Monday morning, wait at least until Wednesday morning of the same week to repeat the same upper-body "push" sequence. This 48-hour rest period gives the primary muscles of your chest, arms, and shoulders time to adequately rebuild, repair, and recover.

Weekly rest:

The second concept of rest is allowing *at least* one day of rest per week from any kind of rigorous exercise. Working out every day of the week will lead to burnout, failure, and injury. Remember, functionally fit firefighters adopt a lifestyle of balance and moderation, and this lifestyle includes balancing exercise with adequate rest.

The amount of rest each individual requires depends on several factors: Age, current fitness level, quality of hydration and nutrition, medical conditions, and pre-existing injuries. For example, a 50-year-old firefighter who has neglected his health, fitness, and nutrition for several years will need to ease back in to working out. A deconditioned firefighter should make it their goal to start exercising three days per week, utilizing the other four days for rest. On the other end of the spectrum, a 25-year-old firefighter who is already possesses an elite level of functional fitness may only require one rest day per week.

As always, functionally fit firefighters listen closely to what their bodies are telling them. If your shoulder's joint or muscles are extremely sore, yet you are planning to do strength training with that same shoulder, consider putting off any workouts that involve that shoulder for a day or two. If the soreness continues or pain develops, don't "work through the pain." Instead, consult a medical professional to have the injury examined.

SLEEP

Firefighters and *sleep*: If you are in the fire service, you will know that these two terms seem contradictory. Whether we are career, paid on-call, or volunteer, we must respond to calls 24 hours a day. This means our sleep is often interrupted, short-lived, or almost nonexistent. At times, it may seem like we survive merely off of caffeine, adrenaline, and pure willpower. However, these are not adequate substitutes for quality sleep.

In addition to physical rest, adequate sleep is perhaps the most important thing we can do to maximize our recovery and improve our functional fitness. The benefits of a good night's sleep are seemingly endless.

WHY IS ADEQUATE SLEEP
IMPORTANT FOR FIREFIGHTERS?

Table 13.1 – BENEFITS OF ADEQUATE SLEEP[10]
Decreased risk of developing heart disease, stroke, hypertension, obesity, diabetes, and kidney disease
Repair of damaged blood vessels
Muscle repair, resulting in muscle strength and mass improvements
Decreased hunger
Improved immune system function
Improved brain function and mental acuity, improved critical thinking, and decision-making abilities
Improved emotional well-being and interpersonal interactions

8 TIPS FOR IMPROVING
THE QUALITY AND QUANTITY OF SLEEP

1. *Exercise... and do it often!* Frequent exercise reduces the time it takes to fall asleep and increases the total duration of a night's sleep. We recommend working up to 5 to 6 days of exercise per week.

2. *Strive to get 7 to 8 hours of sleep per night.* Adjust your bedtime to achieve this goal every night.

3. *Invest in a comfortable bed, pillow, and linens.* The "return on investment" is well worth it.

4. *Avoid using electronic devices immediately before going to sleep.* These include cell phones, tablets, laptops, and the television. They can stimulate the brain instead of allowing it to wind down for sleep.

5. *Sleep in a very dark room with minimal distractions and sound interruptions.* If at the firehouse, turn down or turn off the scanner when sleeping (if possible).

6. *Avoid alcohol, tobacco, and heavy food intake in the evening.* These can cause indigestion and disrupted sleep cycles.

7. *If you need to take a nap, keep it short: 10 to 30 minutes.* Longer naps can make you feel groggy and may make it difficult to fall asleep at night.

8. *If you believe you have chronic sleep problems (e.g. sleep apnea, insomnia, etc.), participate in a sleep study to receive the proper course of treatment.* Unfortunately, sleep disorders are very common to firefighters.

SUCCESS REQUIRES PLANNING

Successful firefighters know the importance of planning and taking a proactive approach to everything that they do—training, preplanning structures, and especially fitness. One of the best ways to incorporate adequate rest days into our weekly workout programs is by proper *planning.*

When planning your weekly workouts, look at the week ahead and give some forethought to the following:

> *How many* total days can you afford to work out?

> According to your schedule, *which* days of the week are you able to work out?

> Do you want to work out while on-duty at the firehouse (if you are a career firefighter)? If so, you may want to schedule "lighter" workouts on your workdays (e.g. flexibility, yoga, core, and endurance-based cardio).

> Do you have a very busy schedule on a certain day that will prohibit you from working out? This is an ideal choice for a *rest day.*

Using these variables as your guide, you can come up with a weekly workout plan. Take a look at the following 5-day sample plan that balances workouts and rest days. A 5-day weekly plan means that you will work out five days and also have two rest days.

> **Monday**: Upper-body (pushes/pulls/carries) strength training

> **Tuesday** (on-duty): Endurance-based cardiovascular training and core strength

> **Wednesday** (on-duty): Rest day

> **Thursday**: Lower-body (lifts or drags) strength training and core strength
> **Friday**: High-intensity interval training and functional yoga or flexibility
> **Saturday**: Total-body strength training circuit (e.g. firefighter circuit)
> **Sunday**: Rest day

Regardless of how you break down your weekly workouts and rest days, make sure you take a proactive approach by planning for each day.

Functionally fit firefighters take their sleep and rest seriously. Using these passive recovery methods will reap huge dividends in optimizing your functional fitness.

WHAT IS ACTIVE RECOVERY?

Active recovery methods utilize recovery techniques that require some level of physical effort or action. We will use active recovery methods in conjunction with passive recovery methods to enhance and accelerate the recovery process in between workouts.

The four techniques of active recovery are:

1. Post-workout cool-down with stretching
2. Self-myofascial release (foam rolling)
3. Massage
4. Hydration and nutrition

WHY IS ACTIVE RECOVERY IMPORTANT FOR FIREFIGHTERS?

Many of us can attest to feeling sore for a couple of days after a very intense workout. This phenomenon is known as *delayed-onset muscle soreness* (DOMS). DOMS is very common after vigorous exercise, especially if we are just getting back into a fitness routine. Some affectionately refer DOMS as "the day after the day after." We typically start to feel sore within 24 hours of exercising, and it usually peaks at 48 hours. By utilizing active recovery methods at the right times, we can decrease our muscle soreness, reduce injury, and accelerate recovery.

HOW TO INCORPORATE ACTIVE RECOVERY INTO YOUR ROUTINES

1. Post-Workout Cool-down and Stretching

Perhaps two of the most beneficial actions that functionally fit firefighters take at the end of their workouts are a *5-minute cool down* followed by a *5-minute stretching routine*. These activities help our bodies (and minds) re-acclimate to their pre-exercise state.

Cool-down routines incorporate light-intensity cardio—*light jog, brisk walk, stationary bike, elliptical, etc.* After the cool-down activity, perform a stretching routine which specifically targets the muscle group(s) you just used in your workout. For example, if you primarily used your lower body for cardiovascular capacity training (e.g. running, sprints, step mill, Jacobs Ladder), use stretches for the lower body—*runner's lunge, child's pose, hamstring stretches, calf stretches, seated or supine hip twists, etc.* Remember to hold static stretches a minimum of 30 seconds and perform 1 to 2 rounds for each stretch.

To refresh your memory on the various types of stretches for each body part, refer to *Chapter 6 – The Big 8: Flexibility.*

2. Self-Myofascial Release (Foam Rolling)

Over the past decade, using a rigid foam roller to alleviate muscle soreness has become increasingly popular. It is particularly beneficial on large muscle groups, specifically those in the legs, hips, and back. Much like we massage a sore shoulder with our hands, foam rolling is a similar form of self-myofascial release (SMR).

Without getting too technical in our explanation of SMR, skeletal muscle tissue is surrounded by a protective covering called *fascia*. When muscles get too inflamed and cause pain or damage, a joint's range of motion can suffer. The direct pressure from SMR is a form of intense massage which "frees up" the fascia and adhesions ("knots") from a muscle. The end result yields greater joint range of motion, flexibility, and decreased pain.

> **" At the end of every workout, dedicate 10 minutes to a cool-down, stretching routine, and foam rolling."**

How Do I Use a Foam Roller?

1. *Choose a commercially made rigid foam roller.* They vary in size and rigidity, but choose one that is approximately 3 feet in length by 6 inches in diameter. If you are just starting to use a foam roller, you may want to choose one that is on the softer side.

2. *With the foam roller on the floor, position your body part (e.g. hip, hamstring, lower back, etc.) over the roller.* You will let gravity do the work. Have 2 to 3 points of direct contact between you and the floor for adequate balance.

3. *Slowly and gently let your muscles roll over the top of the foam roller at a rate of 1 inch per second.* Once you find a specific sore area or "knot," spend 30 seconds applying direct pressure with the foam roller. Move on to other areas after 30 seconds of direct pressure.

4. *Foam rolling can be very uncomfortable.* Use deep breathing to work through the "therapeutic discomfort."

5. *To narrow your SMR focus and specifically target troublesome "knots," use a mini-basketball, tennis ball, racket ball, or lacrosse ball.*

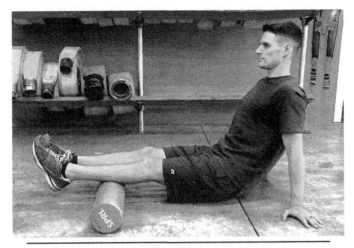

Foam rolling of calf muscles

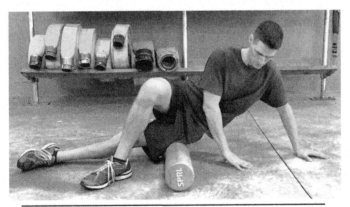

Foam rolling of hips

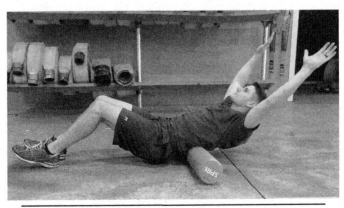

Foam rolling of back

185

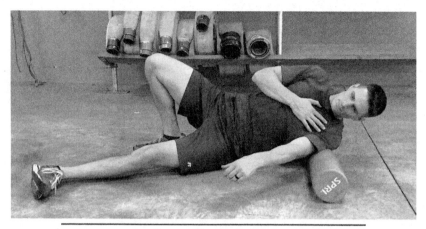

Foam rolling of shoulder

SMR can be used before a workout to warm up and relax overly tight muscles. It can also be used after a workout if you know there are specific muscles you worked extra hard during the workout. If at any point throughout your day you want to use SMR and foam rolling, go for it. There really isn't a wrong time (or limit) to using this active recovery method.

3. Massage

Those of us who have received a massage would probably agree that it is beneficial in rehabilitating the mind, body, and soul. But how does massage affect our functional fitness?

A 10 to 15-minute massage of affected muscles *immediately* after a workout has been shown to speed recovery, improve muscle strength, improve technique, improve body awareness, and reduce injury[11]. Since most of us do not have a personal masseuse available after our workouts, we should perform SMR with a foam roller or by a similar method.

4. Hydration and Nutrition

Although we will discuss how hydration and nutrition specifically relate to firefighter functional fitness the following chapters, we cannot overemphasize the fundamental concept that they greatly affect our *daily* and *long-term* performance, functionality, and recovery.

Functionally fit firefighters know that the quality of their performance directly relates to the quality of their hydration and nutrition. A luxury sports car cannot perform to its maximum potential if we put the wrong kind of fuel in it. Therefore, we must fill our bodies with the best fuels possible. Let's eat right, train hard, and recover properly so we can gain the most benefit from our efforts!

ACTION STEPS:

1. Each week, look at your schedule to plan your workouts and rest days.

2. The next time you perform strength training, allow 48 hours of rest before performing the same type of strength training.

3. Adjust your bedtime to get 7 to 8 hours of sleep per night.

4. After each workout, do a 5 minute cool-down followed by 5 minutes of static stretching and foam rolling.

5. Find or buy a foam roller. Use it before and after workouts to roll out overly tight muscles. You can also use it at any point throughout the day.

6. Continue reading to learn how hydration and nutrition impact your recovery and performance.

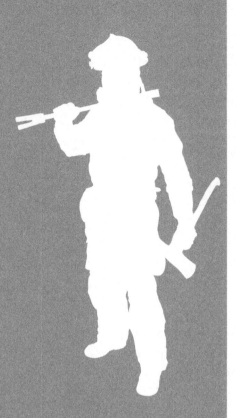

The physical
demands of
firefighting are like
no other sport
or profession.

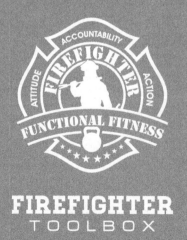

FIREFIGHTER
TOOLBOX

CHAPTER 14
PILLAR 3: HYDRATION

Proper hydration is overlooked by firefighters. The truth is dehydration adversely affects our functional fitness and fireground performance in very significant ways. Most firefighters do not know dehydration also elevates the acute risk of heart attack and stroke—*the primary killers of firefighters*. Chronic dehydration has been linked to cancer and other health-related conditions.

Unfortunately, the majority of firefighters arrive at the firehouse already dehydrated. A 2012 study demonstrated the following regarding firefighter hydration levels prior to training[12]:

> - 31 percent exhibited signs of serious dehydration
> - 46 percent showed signs of significant dehydration
> - 14 percent exhibited minimal dehydration
> - 9 percent were adequately hydrated

According to the study, a staggering *91 percent* of firefighters exhibited some level of dehydration.

What is hydration, and what does it mean to a functionally fit firefighter? In strict terms, hydration is the process of providing an adequate amount of liquid (water) to bodily tissues. Since water makes up 60 percent of our body weight, and we lose water by many means (e.g. sweating, urinating, breathing), it is critical that proper hydration is maintained.

Functionally fit firefighters understand the drastic effects of dehydration on the body during firefighting operations, and they take a proactive approach to preventing these effects. Within this chapter, we will discuss the effects of dehydration, how to adequately hydrate, and the benefits of post-incident rehydration.

WHY IS PROPER HYDRATION IMPORTANT FOR FIREFIGHTERS?

The physical demands of firefighting are like no other sport or profession. Some have compared firefighting to running a marathon in full PPE on a hot day. From physical exertion and environmental heat stress alone, we can sweat out almost *2 liters per hour* while carrying out firefighting operations.

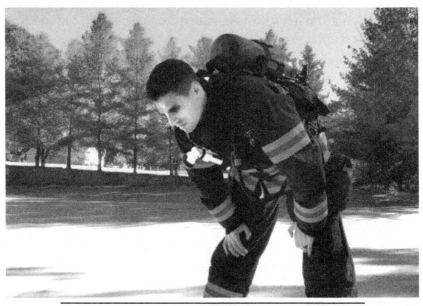

Dehydration is a serious condition for firefighters.

Dehydration has the following physiological effects on our bodies[13]:

- Blood plasma volume decreases
- Blood viscosity (thickness) increases
- Skin blood flow decreases
- Sweating decreases
- Decrease in body heat release and subsequent dissipation
- Core temperature increases
- Muscle glycogen use increases (depleting muscle energy and capacity)

Here is how dehydration negatively effects our physical performance:

> - In laboratory-controlled conditions, VO_2 max (cardiovascular capacity) decreases by 5 percent for a fluid loss of 3 percent body mass. For warm environments (i.e. the fireground), VO_2 max decreases even more. Even for normally hydrated firefighters, environmental heat stress can reduce VO_2 max by 7 percent.
> - The amount of time to exhaustion is reduced by 45 percent for 2.5 percent body weight dehydration. Dehydration reduces the length of time we can effectively perform on the fireground.
> - Dehydration results in both an increased core temperature and a reduction in maximum core temperature tolerance. This is of particular significance since our PPE inhibits heat release and sweat evaporation—compounding the problem of elevated core temperatures.

With regard to heart attack and stroke, dehydration negatively affects our cardiovascular system in six ways[14]:

1. It decreases blood plasma volume.
2. It decreases cardiac output (the amount of blood pumped by the heart every minute).
3. It increases the heart's oxygen demand and metabolic workload because it has to beat faster and more forcefully.
4. It decreases the body's ability to maintain a normal core temperature.
5. It increases blood's viscosity (thickness).
6. It increases the formation of blood clots and blockages.

All of these processes produce a cascade effect that directly contributes to cardiovascular strain. When combining the effects of dehydration with a firefighter's extreme physical workload and hot environment, it is no surprise why we are at such great risk for heart attack and stroke.

HOW CAN I TELL IF I AM DEHYDRATED?
4 SIGNS OF DEHYDRATION

1. **Thirst**: Many of us typically use thirst as an early warning sign of dehydration. However, thirst is not entirely reliable and can actually be a later sign of dehydration. In reality, the very first signs of thirst can mean that the body is already dehydrated.

2. **Dry and sticky mouth and headache**: Following thirst, a dry mouth and headache are signs of more severe dehydration.

3. **Dry and hot skin, low blood pressure, and rapid heart rate**: These symptoms are very late signs of dehydration. Even worse, these symptoms can be signs of heat exhaustion or heat stroke—two very serious, life-threatening conditions for firefighters.

4. **Urine color and volume**: When urinating, if our urine color is dark yellow or orange, has a strong odor, and is relatively small in volume, there is a high probability that we are dehydrated. Certain foods, vitamins, and supplements (beets, asparagus, vitamin B), however, can alter our urine color and odor.

> **"**Caffeinated drinks like coffee, soda, and energy drinks cause us to urinate more frequently, leading to faster onset of dehydration at the fire scene."

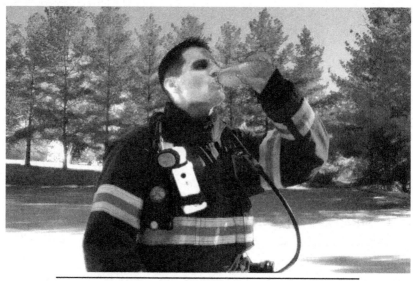

Staying hydrated helps decrease the risk of acute cardiac events and exhaustion.

HOW TO PROPERLY HYDRATE: THE PRP METHOD

For firefighters, proper hydration requires a multifaceted approach. It starts before the incident, it is impacted by firefighter rehabilitation efforts during mitigation, and it requires the flushing of toxins after the incident is over. This is why we want to introduce you to the *PRP Method*. PRP stands for *preparation, rehabilitation,* and *purging*. Functionally fit firefighters use all three to maximize their performance and recovery, and to reduce their risk of heart attack, stroke, injury, and cancer.

1. Preparation

Euhydration is the state of normal body water content or the state of adequate hydration. Unfortunately, many firefighters do not grasp the importance of staying adequately hydrated until the effects of dehydration have already set in. By then, it is too late to quickly recover. Further, what they do drink usually consists of coffee, soda, or energy drinks—all of which typically contain caffeine, a diuretic. Diuretics cause us to urinate more frequently, leading to faster onset of dehydration at the fire scene.

The simple truth is most of us do not consume enough fluids throughout the day, or we consume the wrong kinds of fluids. Many studies show heat stress and hydration level are two physiological responses to firefighting that can increase the chance of a sudden cardiac event. *Functionally fit firefighters know that water is the best choice to maintain euhydration.*

The more proactive our approach is to continuous hydration throughout the day, the less prone we are to dehydration at the fire scene.

HOW MUCH WATER IS ENOUGH TO STAY HYDRATED?

The National Academy of Sports Medicine recommends drinking the following amounts of water each day:

> ➤ *3 liters (approximately 13 cups) for men*
> ➤ *2.2 liters (approximately 9 cups) for women*

These figures are for average-sized, *sedentary* men and women.

Since functionally fit firefighters are performance athletes who regularly experience heat stress and elevated core temperatures, they should aim to exceed these baseline recommendations. Depending on the number of physically demanding alarms a firefighter responds to, their daily fluid intake may far surpass the amounts above.

Functionally fit firefighters are intentional with their hydration efforts throughout the day. If you are someone who likes coffee, try to limit your intake to only one cup in the morning (especially while on-duty). If you are someone who likes soda, energy drinks, and other sugary drinks, limit your consumption to minimal amounts or eliminate them completely. These beverages wreak havoc on blood sugar levels, and typically cause you to eat junk foods and other foods that are high in sodium, unhealthy fats, and calories. What unfortunately results is a repetitive vicious cycle of sugary drinks and salty foods—*not a winning formula for proper hydration and physical performance.*

Like all other aspects of the firefighter functional fitness lifestyle, our daily hydration efforts will use *moderation* and *balance* to achieve euhydration.

10 Tips for Proper Hydration

1. Pick a beverage container (20 to 30-ounce capacity) that has fluid volume markings on the side. Doing so will help you keep track of your daily water intake. Fill it with water and have the goal to drink four or more containers per day.

2. In the morning (and before grabbing a cup of coffee), drink a large glass of water.

3. At or around each meal, drink at least two cups (16 oz.) of water. Drinking plenty of fluids with meals also aids in digestion and prevents overeating.

4. Be proactive about hydration. Drink before thirst sets in.

5. Flavor water with low-calorie, low-sugar additives. Excellent choices include fruits, especially those of the citrus variety (e.g. orange, lime, lemon, and grapefruit). Commercially-made flavor additives are a secondary option.

6. Eat plenty of fruits and vegetables. They are also an excellent source of water, in addition to providing nutrients, vitamins, and fiber.

7. Drink water before, during, and after exercising.

8. Consider electrolyte-replacement drinks during and after strenuous workouts. However, avoid those with high amounts of refined sugars.

9. Drink even more fluids than you would normally consume on hot days (and the day before).

10. Minimize or eliminate your consumption of caffeine, coffee, tea, soda, energy drinks, sugary drinks, and alcohol.

2. Rehabilitation

Rehabilitation is the second step in the PRP Method. Even in cooler climates, firefighters can become easily dehydrated while working at emergency scenes. Not only do we lose fluid volume from sweating but we also excrete electrolytes like sodium, chloride, potassium, magnesium, and calcium. Due to our physical workload, personal protective equipment, and the environmental extremes in which we operate, rehydration during an emergency is critically important.

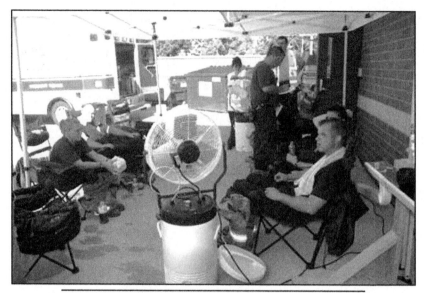

Firefighter rehabilitation is critical for properly rehydrating firefighters during an emergency incident.
Photo courtesy of: Ken Zaccard

At an ongoing incident (e.g. fire, hazmat, rescue, live fire training, etc.), a rehabilitation sector must be established—there are no two ways about it. In the past, firefighter rehabilitation was *recommended*. With the creation of NFPA 1584: *Standard on the Rehabilitation for Members During Emergency Operations and Training Exercises,* firefighter rehabilitation became a *standard* of care. Rehabilitation has been *proven* to decrease the incidence of firefighter injury and death.

The two primary actions for the rehab sector at an emergency scene should be firefighter rehydration and returning a firefighter's core temperature back to normal.

9 STEPS TO OPERATING AN EFFECTIVE REHABILITATION SECTOR

The following steps will help guide you and your fire department in establishing and operating a successful rehabilitation sector at emergency scenes.

1. Locate the rehab area in a relatively controlled environment where firefighters can sit down to rest, well-removed from fireground smoke and scene hazards.

2. Remove firefighters' protective ensembles as soon as possible to allow optimal body heat release and dissipation. Doing so will help a firefighter's core temperature return back to normal.

3. Assess heart rate, blood pressure, respiratory rate, temperature, SpO2 and SpCO (measurement of oxygen and carbon monoxide) as soon as a firefighter enters the rehab sector. Before the firefighter leaves rehab, take a second set of vital signs to ensure that they have returned to normal.

4. Rehydrate and replenish fluids and electrolytes through drinking water and sports drinks. Use those that are low in refined sugars.

5. Treat hyperthermia with passive or active cooling (e.g. wet towels applied to the neck or forearm immersion in cold water).

6. Consider intravenous fluid administration of normal saline (if equipped) for moderate to severe dehydration.

7. Supply calorie replenishment through good carbohydrates (e.g. fruit, granola bars). Avoid consuming refined carbohydrates.

8. Avoid the following: carbonated beverages, caffeine, fast food, and any foods that are high in fat and sugar.

9. Always have a dedicated ambulance available for transport to the emergency room.

After leaving the scene, continue to aggressively rehydrate over the next 12 to 24 hours. In addition to fluid replacement, functionally fit firefighters focus on good food choices—as outlined in *Pillar 4: Nutrition and Lifestyle.*

3. Purging: Rehydration and Cancer Prevention

There is an added benefit to post-incident rehydration: *cancer risk reduction.* As most of us know, cancer is another major epidemic in the fire service. Unfortunately, the words *cancer* and *firefighting* have become synonymous.

Even if we wear the appropriate respiratory equipment at a fire, the carcinogens from smoke are still absorbed through our turnout gear and our skin. After absorption, the carcinogens are transmitted through our blood stream and are eventually deposited into vital organs (e.g. kidneys, liver, etc.). Functionally fit firefighters use euhydration and post-incident rehydration reduce their cancer risk in the following ways[15]:

> Keeping the human body fully hydrated assists in cellular oxygenation. When cells have enough oxygen, they are more cancer resistant.

> Euhydration keeps the immune system functioning properly. This bodily system fights cancer in our cells and keeps it from spreading throughout the body.

> Proper hydration reduces our risk of developing diabetes and obesity. There is a strong link between these two conditions and contracting cancer. Diabetes, cancer, and obesity share many of the same risk factors, and staying hydrated has been shown to decrease the risk of their development.

> After an incident, aggressive rehydration provides our bodies with enough fluid to help flush toxins from our blood, organs, and cells. These toxins are eventually excreted through urine and sweat.

As firefighters, we are regularly forced to push our bodies well beyond their normal physiological capacities. It has been said most people, regardless of occupation, wake up already dehydrated, and the tendency to consume drinks that contribute to dehydration makes the situation even worse. The effects of dehydration, like most other detrimental effects on the firefighter's health, are both *acute* and *chronic*.

Functionally fit firefighters understand the benefits of staying adequately hydrated are seemingly endless. From cancer and disease prevention to optimal performance and recovery, aggressive hydration will help us in all of our functional fitness goals.

Our bodies are not indestructible, but they are resilient. Even if we lacked healthy hydration habits in the past, there is no time like the present to make positive changes. Like other areas of our functional fitness, doing so in "small sips" will lead to greater success.

After reading this chapter, only one question remains: *Who's thirsty?*

ACTION STEPS:

1. Starting today, begin carrying a bottle of water with you at all times.

2. Every morning when you wake up, drink a large glass of water.

3. Begin limiting your intake of caffeinated and sugary drinks. If you drink a lot of soda or coffee, cut back one soda or coffee per day and replace it with water. Once you are used to the adjustment, continue cutting your intake of caffeine and sugary drinks.

4. Find and place a urine color chart in the bathrooms at your fire station. Educate your fellow firefighters on how to read the chart and what to do to stay hydrated.

5. If a rehabilitation sector is not normally established at your fire department's emergency incidents, use NFPA 1584 as a guide to changing the culture.

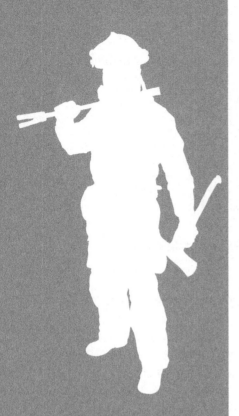

Nutrition isn't simply a two-week program or a fad diet.

It is a way of life.

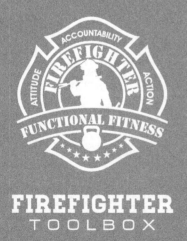

CHAPTER 15

PILLAR 4: NUTRITION AND LIFESTYLE

Disclaimer: The science of nutrition is ever-evolving, and entire books are written on the subject. The principles of nutrition found in this chapter are meant to serve as guidelines for firefighters. The authors are not registered dietitians.

As many fitness enthusiasts have professed before, *you can work out as much as possible, but you can never outwork a poor diet*. There is incredible truth to this statement. As a reader, you could follow all of the fitness guidelines introduced in *Pillar 1: Physical Fitness* and you could exercise every day of the week. However, if your diet consists of nothing but pizza, cheeseburgers, soda, and ice cream, then most of your hard work in the gym will all be for naught.

> ❝ You can work out as much as possible, but you can never outwork a poor diet."

WHAT IS PROPER NUTRITION?

Proper nutrition is about eating the *right foods* in the *right amounts*, so our bodies are provided with all of the *right nutrients* they need for optimal performance. Functionally fit firefighters know that choosing proper nutrition that specifically targets and prevents heart disease will reduce the risk of heart attack, stroke, health-related retirements, and line-of-duty deaths.

> ❝ An ounce of prevention is worth a pound of cure."
> —Benjamin Franklin

Functionally fit firefighters are extremely disciplined, set high personal standards, and take a proactive approach to developing their knowledge, skills, and abilities. In the same vein, functionally fit firefighters must also be proactive when it comes to their nutritional choices.

WHY IS NUTRITION IMPORTANT FOR FIREFIGHTERS?

The difficult but very real truth is that poor nutritional choices are a primary culprit in firefighters developing obesity, diabetes, high cholesterol, hypertension, cancer and other health ailments. All of these disease processes play major roles in firefighters developing cardiovascular disease (CVD).

Let's be honest, *firefighters love to eat*. We all may not agree on tactics, and there are some who do not like to train—*but all firefighters love food*. Unfortunately, this love of food has become a big problem—so much so that more than 70 percent of the American fire service is considered overweight.

> " Proper nutrition is about eating the right foods in the right amounts, so our bodies are provided with all of the right nutrients they need for optimal performance."

As firefighters, we should view our nutrition in the same light as our training: *What we put in is what we get out*. In nutrition and training alike, we will reap what we sow. This is why so many use the cliché: *You are what you eat*. Additionally, both training and nutrition require proper planning, discipline, and attention to detail. The choices we make with our food directly impact our future performance—*not only for tomorrow, but 10, 20, and 30 years down the road*.

HOW TO IMPROVE YOUR NUTRITION

In this chapter, we will present guidelines for healthy nutrition, discuss foods that firefighters should eat less, and give tips for nutritional success. Specifically, we will discuss fats, carbohydrates, proteins, and fiber. Functionally fit firefighters need a balance of each in order to get the most out of their bodies, and this chapter will be the roadmap for your nutritional success.

FATS

Many people hold the unfounded belief that "all fats are bad." In the 1990s, many companies successfully marketed "fat-free" and "low-fat" foods to American consumers who wanted to better their health. The public was led to believe that food fat of any kind was bad for their health because it would cause heart disease and it would cause them to get fat. Fast forward a couple of decades and we now know that this theory is false.

Functionally fit firefighters know fat is an essential macronutrient that the body needs to function properly. It provides energy, helps with cell function, boosts immune system function, and allows certain vitamins to be absorbed into our tissues. Understand however, that fat is high in calories (i.e. 9 calories per gram). Therefore, we must be mindful of how much fat we consume to avoid excessive calorie intake and weight gain. Regardless of the type of macronutrient, taking in more calories than we use on a daily basis leads to weight and body fat gains. As always, *moderation and balance are key.*

There are different types of fat found in the food we consume: unsaturated, saturated, and trans fats. Over the past several decades, Americans were taught that foods with *unsaturated fats* were "good" and *saturated* and *trans fats* were "bad." We will take a closer look at each to clarify some of the confusion.

Which Types of Fats Should We Choose?

Monounsaturated fats improve healthy high-density lipoprotein (HDL) cholesterol (commonly referred to as "good cholesterol") within the blood and keep insulin and blood sugar levels under control for type 2 diabetes.

The best sources of foods with *monounsaturated* fats include:

> Avocados

> Almonds, peanuts, pecans

> Cooking oils (olive, peanut, sesame)

Polyunsaturated fats reduce unhealthy low-density lipoprotein (LDL) cholesterol ("bad cholesterol") and aid in cell development and growth. Polyunsaturated fats contain omega-3 and omega-6 fatty acids. These assist with brain function, arterial contraction and relaxation, lower blood pressure and heart rate, lower triglycerides, reduce the risk of diabetes, and reduce inflammation[16].

The best sources of foods with *polyunsaturated* fats include:

> Walnuts

> Flax seeds and chia seeds

> Leafy vegetables

> Fermented soy foods

> Oily fish (salmon, trout, herring, mackerel, krill oil)

Saturated fat was previously thought to increase the risk of heart disease. Even today, there is debate in the nutritional and medical communities about the health implications of saturated fats. However, numerous studies state saturated fat *reduces* levels of lipoprotein, which is associated with increased risk of heart disease. This type of fat also promotes satiety (fullness), and it has been proven to help lose weight[17].

Saturated fat predominantly comes from animals and animal products, but it is also found in some plant-based sources.

The best sources of foods with *saturated* fats include:

> Naturally raised, grass-fed organic meats

> Eggs

> Organic, raw dairy (e.g. butter ... yes, butter!)

> Coconut oil

Avoid foods with saturated fats that have been heavily processed (e.g. hot dogs, pepperoni, commercially-made meat sticks, etc.).

Which Types of Fats Should We Avoid?

Trans fats increase our risk of cardiovascular disease by lowering healthy HDL cholesterol and raising unhealthy LDL cholesterol levels. Additionally, high intake of trans fats can lead to the development of diabetes[18]. Trans fats are in foods that have partially hydrogenated vegetable oil, shortening, and some dairy fat. They may include:

> - Anything fried and battered (French fries, doughnuts, fried chicken, onion rings)
> - Anything with shortening (biscuits, bread rolls, crackers, cookies, muffins, pie crust, cakes, icing)
> - Margarine spreads and sticks
> - Some ice cream, milkshakes, and frozen or creamy beverages
> - Butter-flavored microwave popcorn

CARBOHYDRATES

Carbohydrates are another macronutrient essential to our bodies. Contrary to the popular "low-carb" and "no-carb" diet fads from the early 2000s, *not all carbohydrates are bad*. Quality carbohydrates provide glucose to our bodies which then is converted into energy. These carbohydrates also deliver fiber, nutrients, vitamins, and minerals[19].

WHICH TYPES OF CARBOHYDRATES SHOULD WE CHOOSE?

We want to feed our bodies carbohydrates that digest *slowly*. These are *natural* carbohydrates, preferably those with a low to moderate glycemic index. Their slow metabolism helps us stay satiated longer and helps us to avoid dramatic spikes and drops in blood sugar. The frequent "blood sugar rollercoaster" is bad for our bodies because it eventually leads to insulin resistance, diabetes, *and* heart disease[20].

The following food choices contain quality carbohydrates with a low to moderate glycemic index:

> **Whole grains**: Oatmeal (steel-cut or old-fashioned, *not instant*), whole wheat, farro, millet, quinoa, barley, brown rice (*not white*), rye, spelt, and wild rice
> **Fruits**: Apples, cherries, bananas, peach, and citrus fruits (oranges, grapefruit)
> **Vegetables**: Legumes (peas, beans, and lentils) corn, broccoli, tomatoes, carrots, and sweet potatoes (twice the fiber content of white potatoes)

WHICH TYPES OF CARBOHYDRATES SHOULD WE AVOID OR ELIMINATE?

Functionally fit firefighters minimize or eliminate their consumption of *refined carbohydrates*. These carbohydrates have been processed in a way that removes the whole grain. The processing removes healthy nutrients, vitamins, fiber, and healthy oils. They also cause our blood sugar to spike and drop very quickly, which is unhealthy for our metabolism and insulin levels.

The following foods are refined carbohydrates or they have a high glycemic index—both of which should be *minimally consumed*:

> **Foods with white flour**: White bread, white pasta, bagels, muffins, and pancake or waffle mixes (unless "whole grains" is the first ingredient listed, it is made primarily from refined carbohydrates)
> **White rice, instant rice, instant oatmeal, and sugary cereals**
> **White potatoes** (fried *and* baked)
> **Most snacks and junk foods**: Crackers, pretzels, and chips
> **Sugar-added foods**: Cookies, candy, ice cream, and pies
> **Sweeteners**: White and brown sugar*, high-fructose corn syrup, honey, maple and agave syrup
> **Sugary drinks**: Soda, sweetened tea, and energy drinks
> **Alcohol**

Sugar is like kryptonite to firefighters. Excessive intake of sugar not only leads to obesity, diabetes, and heart disease, studies have demonstrated that it also increases the risk of contracting cancer.

Start keeping track of how much sugar you consume on a daily basis—you will be very surprised. Whether it is one less soda or one less cookie per day, any reduction in sugar will be beneficial.

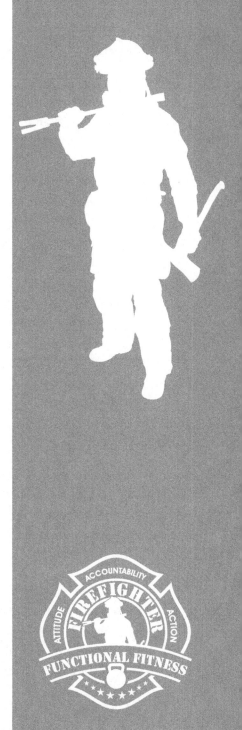

FIREFIGHTER
TOOLBOX

PROTEINS

The "nutrition experts" of 1990s told us to steer clear of fats. In the early 2000s, they wanted us to be carb-free. Fast-forward to current day, and it seems that *protein* is all the rage. The supplement industry is extremely lucrative due in large part to protein supplement sales. These companies try to lead us to believe our bodies need as much protein as possible if we want to get stronger (or build mass). However, functionally fit firefighters know 10 to 35 percent of daily calories should come from protein[21].

As firefighters, we love our protein. If we cook hamburgers, we tend to make huge patties, throw a couple slices of cheese on top, and then add a couple slices of bacon. When we order a pizza, the "more meat, more cheese" mindset usually wins. Unfortunately, excessive protein intake (especially from the wrong sources), is harmful to our bodies. Too much protein can cause kidney disease, weight gain, body fat gain, dehydration, cancer, and shortened life expectancy. Again, we cannot overemphasize the concept of balance and moderation when it comes to our overall nutrition.

Which Types of Proteins Should We Choose?

For all types of animal protein, we should choose the most natural option possible. Animals that have been raised in natural conditions provide meat that has higher nutritional values. Whenever possible, choose *organic, grass fed, free-range, cage-free, preservative-free, and hormone-free* options.

> - **Poultry**: Grilled or baked, *not breaded and fried*
> - **Fish**: Salmon, trout, and herring (preferably wild caught, not farm-raised)
> - **Beef, pork, and lamb**
> - **Game meats**: Venison, buffalo, elk, etc.
> - **Nuts**: Almonds, peanuts, walnuts, and cashews (raw or lightly salted, and non-roasted, if possible)
> - **Legumes**: Beans, lentils, chickpeas, soybeans, and tofu
> - **Low-fat Greek yogurt**

Which Types of Proteins Should We Eat Less?

As mentioned in the Fats section, we should reduce or eliminate our consumption of meat products that have been

> To get *lean* you must eat *clean* and train *mean*."

overly-processed (e.g. hot dogs, meat sticks, pepperoni, etc.). Also, avoid eating meats that have been fried in unhealthy trans-fat oils.

FIBER

When we discussed carbohydrates, we mentioned the importance of consuming dietary fiber. There are two types of fiber: soluble and insoluble fiber. *Why are these fibers important?* **Soluble fiber** slows down digestion and promotes satiety. **Insoluble fiber** helps with digestion and keeps our gastrointestinal system moving[22].

Eating foods that are rich in fiber benefits our body in several ways:

- Reduces the risk of cardiovascular disease (heart attack and stroke)
- Reduces the risk of developing diabetes by controlling blood sugar (slows the rate of carbohydrate digestion and absorption)
- Promotes weight loss by increasing satiety
- Prevents constipation

The United States Food and Drug Administration (FDA) recommends men and women consume 38 grams and 25 grams of dietary fiber each day, respectively.

Fiber-Rich Foods

- **Fresh fruit**: Pears, apples, raspberries, bananas, blueberries, oranges, and strawberries
- **Dried fruit**: Prunes, dried figs, raisins, and dried apricots
- **Vegetables**: Artichoke hearts, pea varieties, leafy greens (spinach, mustard, collard), corn, brussels sprouts, broccoli, onions, green beans, and sweet potatoes

> **Legumes**: Chickpeas, pea varieties, lentils, and beans
> **Nuts and Seeds**: Flaxseed, chia seeds, almonds, pistachios, pumpkin seeds, and sesame seeds
> **Whole Grains**: Oatmeal (steel-cut or old-fashioned, not instant), oat bran, popcorn, whole wheat, farro, millet, quinoa, brown rice (not white), rye, spelt, and wild rice

CANCER-FIGHTING FOODS

In additional to the cardiovascular epidemic, *cancer* is the other major health problem that is confronting firefighters. For certain types of cancers, firefighters face a 50 to 100 percent increased risk as compared to the general population. Many firefighters tend to solely focus on "wearing their air" and washing their gear for cancer protection, but we can also greatly decrease our cancer risks by eating the right foods, controlling our weight, and preventing diabetes.

" Firefighters can greatly decrease their cancer risks by eating the right foods, controlling their weight, and by preventing diabetes."

In the following table, you will notice that all of the foods listed are *natural* foods: fruits, vegetables, nuts, whole grains, and more. Many of them are foods we have already presented in this chapter. Balance these foods with other aspects of a healthy lifestyle (e.g. exercise, hydration, weight control, and tobacco abstention) to proactively prevent cancer.

Table 15.1 – A TO Z LIST OF CANCER-FIGHTING FOODS [23]
Apples
Berries (blueberries, blackberries, raspberries, acai)
Broccoli
Carrots
Cauliflower
Cherries
Chili Peppers
Citrus Fruits (oranges/lemons)
Coffee
Cranberries
Flaxseed
Garlic
Grapes
Grapefruit
Leafy Greens (kale, spinach)
Legumes (beans, peas, lentils)
Melons
Mushrooms
Nuts
Onions
Papayas
Pomegranates
Soy
Squash (Winter)
Strawberries
Tea
Tomatoes
Walnuts
Whole grains

25 TIPS FOR NUTRITIONAL SUCCESS

1. **Don't confuse *proper nutrition* with "going on a diet."** Many diets fail because they are too restrictive and unrealistic. Proper nutrition, by contrast, is how we provide appropriate *nourishment* for our bodies. Nutrition isn't a two-week program or a fad diet—*it is a way of life*.

2. **Go natural**. As a rule of thumb, choose natural, minimally-processed, preservative-free foods. Ask yourself: *Would my ancestors from hundreds of years ago eat the same foods that I am eating? Would they even recognize the foods that I am eating?* If the answer is "no," go a more natural route with your food choices.

3. **Write down your nutrition and fitness goals**. By documenting these goals, the more likely you will commit to them. Use the SMART method of goal-setting: make them *specific, measurable, attainable, relevant*, and *time-bound*. Keep track of your progress and reward yourself for reaching specific milestones.

4. **Don't obsess about a number on the scale**. Remember: *Firefighter Functional Fitness* is not about getting "washboard abs" or 5 percent body fat. If you are overweight and want to lose a few pounds, lose enough weight until you are satisfied with your *level of performance*. If you truly want to lose weight, remember there are no shortcuts: *To **get lean** you must **eat clean** and **train mean***. For more tips on how to lose weight, read Chapter 22: *25 Frequently Asked Questions*.

5. **Think *quality* over *quantity***. By eating the *right* foods (and not necessarily *less* food), performance and body composition will drastically improve. As a rule of thumb, always pick fresh, natural foods over chemically processed foods. Processed foods are usually higher in calories, unnatural preservatives, and other artificial ingredients.

6. **Take baby steps**. Making small, positive nutrition choices *consistently* will produce big dividends (e.g. one less soda per day, one extra glass of water, one extra piece of fruit or serving of vegetables, etc.).

7. **Try new foods**. Every week, try a healthy food listed above that you haven't eaten before. Use the Internet to research

different ways to prepare it. You might be surprised at the results.

8. **Keep healthy foods visible and readily accessible**. The more we keep good food choices in plain sight, the more likely we are to actually eat them.

9. **What you don't see will help you**. Keep foods you should avoid "out of sight, out of mind." Put them in places that are more difficult to access. The less we see them, the less opportunities we have to be reminded about them.

10. **Plan!** This is incredibly important for the unpredictable schedule that firefighters have. Due to call volume, we usually make food choices based on what is convenient at the time. This leads us to choose foods that are high in bad fats, calories, and preservatives (fast food and pizza are the usual suspects). Plan and cook three healthy dinners per week. Make enough to have leftovers for lunch the next day.

11. **Eat slowly**. Firefighters tend to eat too quickly because we are accustomed to getting a call at any moment. When we eat in a controlled, slow manner, we are better able to sense when we are getting full.

12. **Occasionally indulge**. If you are going to eat something indulgent (pizza, ice cream, fast food, etc.), limit your portion sizes. Treat yourself once a week to these types of foods, but avoid consuming them on a daily basis.

13. **Eat at home**. Instead of "eating out," prepare as many meals as possible at home and at the fire house. In these environments, you have ultimate control over the choice of ingredients and how your food is prepared.

14. **When eating at a restaurant, be disciplined in your choices**. Instead of a bacon cheeseburger, choose a turkey burger with a whole grain bun. Instead of french fries, choose a baked potato or sweet potato (without the bacon and sour cream). Portions at restaurants are usually very large. Therefore, eat half of your meal at the restaurant, and bring home the other half for a separate meal.

15. **Go "on the record."** Keep track of what you eat, specifically through measuring it and writing it down. There are numerous food diary apps for smartphones (e.g. My Fitness Pal, MyPlate Calorie Tracker, etc.), or use the good old-fashioned paper journal.

16. **Spice it up**. To add maximum flavor without adding maximum calories and sodium, use hot (chili) sauces and citrus (i.e. lemon, lime) on your favorite foods.

17. **Measure out snacks and other portions**. When snacking on foods like chips, portion out a specific amount into a bowl. Close up the bag and put it back in the pantry. When we eat snack foods directly out of their containers, we tend to eat much larger portion sizes.

18. **Use smaller plates to encourage portion control**. Research has shown reducing the size of our plates reduces the overall amount that we eat.

19. **Only eat when you are truly hungry.** Boredom leads to grazing and eating when you are not hungry. Stay busy, distract yourself with other activities—exercise, read, or do hands-on training. Do your best to stay out of the kitchen.

20. **Eat smaller, more frequent meals**. Instead of two or three very large meals, eat three medium meals with three healthy snacks. Overeating makes us feel bloated, results in excessive calorie consumption, and causes blood sugar levels to rapidly spike and drop. Avoid skipping meals; doing so causes excessive hunger, which then leads to overeating.

21. **Get expert advice**. Meet with a personal trainer and dietician to come up with a custom plan that will lead to nutritional success.

22. **Consider sweet treat alternatives**. If you desire a sweet treat after a meal (*and who doesn't*), consider a piece of low-sugar gum. Gum is usually 5 calories per stick, it can satisfy your sweet tooth, and it helps clean your teeth. An alternative sweet treat is a piece of dark chocolate.

23. **Being successful with your nutrition requires PRIDE** *(Personal Responsibility In Daily Effort)*. No one can do it for you. It requires an "all-in" attitude, and it is a daily commitment.

24. **Use the buddy system**. With a friend or with your firehouse crew, use an accountability system to keep each other honest about what you eat. Inspire a little healthy competition by issuing nutritional challenges to each other. If possible, eat healthy meals together, work out together,

set goals together, encourage each other, and share fitness successes.

25. **Practice *everything in moderation above all else*.** Nutrition and functional fitness require balance and moderation. Avoid extremes like "always" and "never" in your food choices.

ACTION STEPS:

1. Each week, implement 1 to 2 tips from the *25 Tips for Nutritional Success*.

2. Remove unhealthy snack foods from plain view—both in the fire station and at home.

3. Learn the difference between monounsaturated, polyunsaturated, saturated, and trans fats. Reduce or eliminate your consumption of foods with trans fats.

4. Inventory your snack cabinet at home and at the fire station. Reduce or eliminate those foods that are high in refined carbohydrates and sugar.

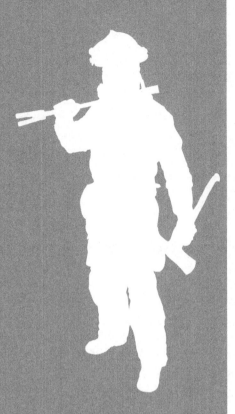

The best time for you to work out has nothing to do with a clock.

It is when you feel most motivated to work out.

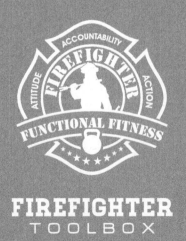

FIREFIGHTER
TOOLBOX

CHAPTER 16

WORKOUT PROGRAMMING: PUTTING IT ALL TOGETHER

Throughout this book, we have discussed numerous functional fitness topics. More importantly, we have provided several examples of how to make your fitness training functional through *The Big 8* concept.

Now that you know what *Firefighter Functional Fitness* is and why it is important, we will dive deeper by giving you guidance on how to put everything into action. This chapter will teach you how to program your daily and weekly workouts. *Programming* is a fitness term used to describe how to set up or plan your daily and weekly workout routines.

As a disclaimer, we will let you know that it is impossible for us to provide *every* variation of *every* workout routine in a single book. If we did, this book would be never-ending.

At its core, workout programming for *Firefighter Functional Fitness* blends all aspects of *The Big 8*: Core, Cardiovascular Capacity, Flexibility, Pushing, Pulling, Lifting, Carrying, and Dragging. Within our weekly workouts, we will also balance principles that we have discussed in *Pillar 2: Recovery and Rest*.

LEVELS OF FITNESS CONDITIONING

The very first step in workout programming is to know our starting points and our individual levels of fitness. That is to say, we must address the fact that all of us are at different levels of fitness conditioning.

> " Firefighter Functional Fitness is not a destination, it is a continuous journey to become the most functionally fit version of yourself!"

Conditioning is a term used to describe a person's level of fitness. A well-conditioned, functionally fit firefighter is a firefighter who regularly incorporates all aspects of The 4 Pillars and The Big 8 into their lifestyle. On the other hand, a deconditioned firefighter could be someone who rarely or never exercises and neglects their hydration and nutrition.

There are several components that combine to determine a firefighter's functional fitness conditioning level:

> - Muscular strength, endurance, and power
> - Core stability
> - Balance
> - Flexibility
> - Cardiovascular capacity

If we are honest with ourselves, each of us could subjectively rate our individual functional fitness conditioning levels. That is to say, each of us would be able to generally categorize ourselves as either *"out-of-shape," "average,"* or *"in-shape."*

The Firefighter Functional Fitness Performance Assessment

In order to obtain a more objective and realistic picture of your current overall level of functional fitness, we designed the *Firefighter Functional Fitness Performance Assessment* to help determine whether you are at *Level 1* (deconditioned), *Level 2* (average), or *Level 3* (well-conditioned).

The assessment is designed to be a simple, yet comprehensive tool to evaluate the five functional fitness conditioning variables listed above. There are other fitness assessments that can be used to better quantify cardiovascular capacity (i.e. VO_2 max), but they require expensive equipment and the direct supervision of a fitness professional. Our assessment, on the other hand, can be completed by an individual, with minimal equipment.

Directions: Complete each station as written, with one minute rest intervals in between each station. As with all other types of exercise, make sure that you are medically-cleared for physical activity by your medical professional.

FIREFIGHTER FUNCTIONAL FITNESS PERFORMANCE ASSESSMENT

Station	Level 1	Level 2	Level 3
Push-Ups (Total Reps in 1 Minute)	< 10 (Male) < 7 (Female)	11–44 (Male) 8–34 (Female)	< 45 (Male) < 35 (Female)
Air Squats (Total Reps in 1 Minute)	< 15	16–29	< 30
Standard Plank (Total Duration)	< 30 seconds	31–59 seconds	< 60 seconds
Balance on One Leg, Standing (Both Sides 15 seconds)	Raised foot touches ground	Moderate difficulty (Wobbling)	No difficulty
Sit-and-Reach Hamstring Stretch	Unable to reach toes	Able to reach toes	Can reach past toes
YMCA 3-Minute Step Test*	See charts below	See charts below	See charts below

*The *YMCA 3-Minute Step Test* is used to determine an individual's cardiovascular capacity rating. It measures how quickly one's heart rate recovers after physical activity. Follow these steps to complete the test:

1. Step up and down from a 12-inch platform at a rate of 96 steps per minute. Use a metronome to stay on pace. Metronome apps can be downloaded on smartphones.
2. Perform this test for a total of 3 minutes.

3. Within 5 seconds of finishing the test, record your recovery pulse rate for a total of 60 seconds. To obtain your pulse rate, place your index and middle fingers on your inner wrist by your thumb. Use gentle pressure.

4. Locate your recovery pulse rate on the charts below to determine your current cardiovascular capacity rating. "Very Poor to Poor" coincides with Level 1, "Below Average to Above Average" coincides with Level 2, and "Good to Excellent" coincides with Level 3 on the Firefighter Functional Fitness Performance Assessment.

YMCA Heart Rate Chart (MEN): Based on age.

	18-25	26-35	36-45	46-55	56-65	65+
Excellent	50-75	51-76	49-76	56-82	60-77	59-81
Good	79-84	79-85	80-88	87-93	86-94	87-92
Above Average	88-93	88-94	92-88	95-101	97-100	94-102
Average	95-100	96-102	100-105	103-111	103-109	104-110
Below Average	102-107	104-110	108-113	113-119	111-117	114-118
Poor	111-119	114-121	116-124	121-126	119-128	121-126
Very Poor	124-157	126-161	130-163	131-159	131-154	130-151

YMCA Heart Rate Chart (WOMEN): Based on age.

	18-25	26-35	36-45	46-55	56-65	65+
Excellent	52-81	58-80	51-84	63-91	60-92	70-92
Good	85-93	85-92	89-96	95-101	97-103	96-101
Above Average	96-102	95-101	100-104	104-110	106-111	104-111
Average	104-110	104-110	107-112	113-118	113-118	116-121
Below Average	113-120	113-119	115-120	120-124	119-127	123-126
Poor	122-131	122-129	124-132	126-132	129-135	128-133
Very Poor	135-169	134-171	137-169	137-171	141-174	135-155

When performing the assessment, it is likely that you will fall under different levels for different stations. For example: An individual with elite muscular strength but poor flexibility, balance, and cardiovascular capacity, may fall under *Level 3* in the push-up and air squat stations while placing in *Level 1* for the balance, flexibility, and YMCA 3-Minute Step Test stations. The long-term goal for every functionally fit firefighter is to reach *Level 3* in each station of the assessment.

Once you have completed your individual *Firefighter Functional Fitness Performance Assessment*, the next step is to establish a workout program that suits your needs. In this chapter, we will provide guidelines and sample programs for each of the three levels based on The Big 8. Regardless of your current level of functional fitness, remember all of us are works in progress. *Firefighter Functional Fitness* is not a destination, it is a continuous journey to become the most functionally fit version of yourself!

HOW TO PROGRAM WEEKLY WORKOUTS

After you have determined your fitness conditioning level, the next step is to determine how many days per week you will commit to exercising. Follow these guidelines:

Level 1

If you are in this category, we encourage you to start exercising 3 days per week. Use the 3-day weekly program for a total of 4 to 6 weeks until you start to see improvements in your functional fitness. At the end of 4 to 6 weeks, repeat the *Firefighter Functional Fitness Performance Assessment* to see if you are ready to graduate to the next level.

Level 2

If you are in this category, exercise 4 days per week. Use the 4-day weekly program for a total of 4 to 6 weeks until you start to see improvements in your functional fitness. At the end of 4 to 6 weeks, repeat the *Firefighter Functional Fitness Performance Assessment* to see if you are ready for *Level 3*.

Level 3

If you are in this category, it is likely that you already exercise 5 to 6 days per week. Continue on this path to optimizing your fireground performance. The ultimate goal for functionally fit firefighters is to dedicate 5 to 6 days of exercise per week. Later in this chapter, we will provide you with 3-day, 4-day, and 5 to 6-day sample programs.

Firefighter Functional Fitness uses workout programming by "day of the week" because it incorporates and balances all areas of The Big 8. Keep in mind that integrating rest days is crucial to improving functional fitness and for injury prevention, avoiding fatigue, and burnout.

By programming workouts correctly, there will be no need to spend countless hours in the gym. As functionally fit firefighters, we must also be sure we do not overexert ourselves, especially when working out while on-duty. Whatever we decide, the most important thing to remember is our training should be effective, efficient, safe, and *functional*. Keeping things simple is a good approach—*just don't confuse simple with easy!*

> **Keeping things simple is a good approach—just don't confuse simple with easy!"**

As we develop our routines, one of the best parts about *Firefighter Functional Fitness* is most workouts will have a primary focus, but they may simultaneously address closely-related functional areas. For example, a "push workout" for upper and lower body can also incorporate core strength, cardiovascular capacity training, lifts, carries, drags, etc. You are only limited by your imagination when you combine exercises from The Big 8.

WHAT ARE THE KEY ELEMENTS OF A *FIREFIGHTER FUNCTIONAL FITNESS* WEEKLY PROGRAM?

Core Strength Training

> - 2 to 4 times per week
> - 10 to 30 minutes per session
> - To be combined with another modality (e.g. flexibility, cardio, strength)

Cardiovascular Capacity Training

> - 3 or more times per week
> - One HIIT session, one EBCT session, and one firefighter circuit training session
> - 30 to 60 minutes per session, depending on current conditioning level and intensity of activity

Flexibility Training

> - *Dynamic stretching* during warm-ups
> - *Static stretching* during cool-downs
> - One or more *long flexibility* training per week (e.g. 30 minutes of functional yoga)

Functional Strength Training

> - 3 or more times per week (one upper-body session, one lower-body session, and one total-body session)
> - 20 to 32 total sets per session (e.g. upper-body push-pull session: 10 to 16 sets of pushing exercises, 10 to 16 sets of pulling exercises)
> - Upper-body sessions combining pushing, pulling, and carrying exercises are ideal
> - Lower-body sessions combining lifting, carrying, and dragging exercises are ideal
> - Total-body sessions combining all elements of The Big 8

FUNCTIONAL FITNESS TERMS

As we move into programming levels, there are some terms and acronyms you will need to understand:

> **AMRAP**: "As many repetitions as possible" within a given timeframe. This is a conditioning-based approach to exercise that primarily benefits cardiovascular capacity. *Example: Push-ups AMRAP for 60 seconds.*

> **Complex**: A complex combines a series of individual exercises for the purpose of completing them in their entirety without stopping for a break. They can be repeated numerous times, depending on one's goals and personal preference. Complexes are often used in Russian kettlebell training. Complexes are high-intensity training sessions that focus on improving cardiovascular capacity. *Example of a kettlebell complex: Complete five double swings, five double snatches, five double clean and press, five double front squat, and five push-ups on the bells.*

> **Fitness Circuit/Circuit Challenge**: A fitness circuit connects a series of individual exercises together in a station-by-station format. The participant moves from one to the next, and completes an exercise at each station. Circuit challenges add competition to the mix either by adding a time constraint or goal, by adding weight or other physical restrictions to the participant, by including specific skills into the circuit, by requiring the participant to complete the circuit more than once, or any combination thereof. These are particularly useful for *Firefighter Functional Fitness* because we can incorporate common fireground skills with a fitness element. An example of a firefighter functional fitness circuit is 1) supply hose drag for 50 feet, 2) overhead sledgehammer strike for 20 reps, 3) stair climb for two stories, 4) firefighter crawl for 50 feet, and 5) Hose section hoist with rope 25 feet. You would repeat this circuit 3 to 6 rounds.

> **Rep**: Abbreviation of "repetition." *Example: 10 reps of squats per set, 4 sets will yield 40 total reps.*

> **Superset**: Alternating two complimentary *or* antagonistic exercises into a back and forth "mini-circuit" with minimal or no rest in between each. Example: Complete three rounds of

push-ups and pull-ups—going back and forth between each exercise. Or one could alternate sets of upper-body and lower-body strength training exercises.

LEVEL 1: THE 3-DAY WEEKLY PROGRAM

If the *Firefighter Functional Fitness Performance Assessment* placed you at *Level 1*, you will begin by doing the 3-day weekly program.

Again, it is our ultimate goal to blend all aspects of The Big 8: core strength, cardiovascular capacity, flexibility, push, pull, lift, carry, and drag. At the end of this chapter, we have included all of the exercises, movements, and stretches from The Big 8 for you to pick and choose from. Substitute different exercises from each category to keep your workouts interesting and constantly changing.

Perform the following 3-Day Weekly program for 4 to 6 weeks, then repeat the performance assessment to see if you are ready to proceed to the next level.

> **Day 1**: Firefighter circuit (HIIT cardiovascular capacity and strength training) and core strength training
> **Day 2**: Rest day
> **Day 3**: Lower-body strength training and flexibility
> **Day 4**: Rest day
> **Day 5**: Cardiovascular capacity (EBCT) and upper-body strength training
> **Day 6**: Rest day
> **Day 7**: Rest day

Each of the workouts should take approximately 45 to 60 minutes to complete.

Day 1: Firefighter Circuit (HIIT* & Strength Training) and Core			
Sequence	**Exercise**	**Reps/Duration**	**Rest Period**
Warm-Up	Jogging, Stationary Bike, Stair Climber, etc.	5 minutes	N/A
Firefighter Circuit** (2–3 Rounds)	Overhead Sledgehammer (Striking Tire)	10 reps with each arm leading, 30 second duration	30 seconds
	Stair Climb	2 stories, up and down, for 30 seconds	30 seconds
	Tire/Dummy/Supply Hose Drag (100–200 lbs.)	50 feet	30 seconds
	Firefighter Crawl	50 feet	30 seconds
	Farmer's Carry with Heavy Equipment (Saws or Tools)	50 feet	30 seconds
	Hose Hoist With Rope (50-foot Section of 3-inch Hose)	30 seconds	30 seconds
Core Circuit (1–2 Rounds)	Supine Leg Lifts	10 reps	N/A
	Standard or Elbow Plank	30 seconds	N/A
	Side Plank	30 seconds (both sides)	N/A
	Bridge Pose	30 seconds	N/A
	Side Bend (Weighted or Unweighted)	10 reps (both sides)	N/A
Flexibility Circuit (1–2 Rounds)	Supine Hamstring Stretch	30 seconds (both legs)	N/A
	Child's Pose	30 seconds	N/A
	Runner's Lunge Stretch	30 seconds (both legs)	N/A
	Butterfly Stretch	30 seconds	N/A
	Overhead Tricep Stretch	30 seconds (both arms)	N/A
Cool-Down	Walking/Jogging (Light Cardio)	5 minutes	N/A
Foam Rolling	Legs, Hips, Back, Shoulders	5 minutes	N/A

**High-intensity interval training requires heart rate to be at or above 85 percent of maximum heart rate. If unable to monitor heart rate, push yourself to near-maximum exertion during the high-intensity intervals.

**For the firefighter circuit, consider the following stages of increasing difficulty:

Stage 1: Wear gym attire (shorts and t-shirt) only.

Stage 2: Add turnout coat and pants, boots, helmet, and gloves.

Stage 3: Add SCBA cylinder.

Stage 4: Add SCBA cylinder, SCBA mask on, and breathe air from cylinder.

At *Level 1*, execute the firefighter circuit at Stage 1 for two weeks, then Stage 2 for the next two weeks, and then Stage 3 or 4 for the final two weeks.

Day 2: Rest

Day 3: Lower-Body Strength and Flexibility Training

Sequence	Exercise	Reps/Duration	Rest Period
Warm-Up	Jogging, Stationary Bike, Stair Climber, etc.	5 minutes	N/A
Lower-Body Circuit (2–3 rounds)	Barbell Squats or Double Kettlebell Front Squats	10 reps	60 seconds
	Medicine Ball Squat Press and Throw	10 reps	60 seconds
	Barbell or Kettlebell Deadlifts	10 reps	60 seconds
	Lunges (Weighted or Unweighted)	10 reps (both legs)	60 seconds

Sequence	Exercise	Reps/Duration	Rest Period
Cool-Down	Light Cardio	5 minutes	N/A
Flexibility/ Yoga Circuit* (2 Rounds)	Supine Hamstring Stretch	30 seconds	N/A
	Calf Stretch Against Wall	30 seconds (both legs)	N/A
	Runner's Lunge Stretch	30 seconds (both legs)	N/A
	Happy Baby Pose	30 seconds	N/A
	Pigeon Pose	30 seconds	N/A
	Chest Opener With Dowel Rod	10 reps	N/A
	Downward Dog	30 seconds	N/A
	Cat and Cow Poses (Alternating)	30 seconds	N/A
	Baby Cobra Pose	30 seconds	N/A
Foam Rolling	Legs and Hips	5 minutes	N/A

*For an abundance of free yoga instructional videos and flexibility training routines, go to *YouTube.com* and search "beginner's or basic yoga for flexibility" or "flexibility training." There are also many gyms that offer basic yoga classes.

Day 4: Rest

Day 5: Cardiovascular Capacity (EBCT*) and Upper-Body Strength			
Sequence	**Exercise**	**Reps/Duration**	**Rest Period**
Warm-Up	Jogging, Stationary Bike, Stair Climber, etc.	5 minutes	N/A
Medium of Your Choice* (Moderate Intensity)	Stair Climbing	30 minutes	N/A
	Swimming	30 minutes	N/A
	Cycling or Stationary Bike	30 minutes	N/A
	Running/Treadmill	30 minutes	N/A
	Rowing	30 minutes	N/A
	Elliptical Machine	30 minutes	N/A
Upper-Body Circuit (2–3 Rounds)	Push-Ups	AMRAP (as many reps as possible)	60 seconds
	Pull-Ups	AMRAP	60 seconds
	Dips	AMRAP	60 seconds
	Inverted Rows	AMRAP	60 seconds
	Standing Overhead Press (Dumbbells or Kettlebells)	10 reps	60 seconds
	Angled Cable Row or Bent-Over Row	10 reps	60 seconds
	Sled Push With Gym Mat	50 FEET	60 seconds
	Kneeling Cable Row (Hose Pulling or Hooking Ceiling Simulation)	10 reps (Both Sides)	60 seconds
Cool-Down/ Flexibility	Static Stretching for Upper Body	5 minutes	N/A
Foam Rolling	Upper Body and Back	5 minutes	N/A

*Endurance-based cardiovascular training (EBCT) requires a heart rate at 70 to 85 percent of maximum heart rate. The exercise choices for EBCT can be broken down into shorter durations and mixed for a total of 30 to 60 minutes in one workout session. As long as one's heart rate stays in the 70 to 85 percent range, any exercise medium can be used for EBCT—traditional "cardio," strength training, yoga, etc. If unable to monitor heart rate, push yourself enough to elevate your respiratory rate moderately (but you should still be able to speak in full sentences).

Day 6: Rest

Day 7: Rest

LEVEL 2: THE 4-DAY WEEKLY PROGRAM

If the *Firefighter Functional Fitness Performance Assessment* placed you at *Level 2*, you will begin by doing the 4-day weekly program.

Perform the following 4-day weekly program for 4 to 6 weeks, then repeat the performance assessment to see if you are ready to proceed to the next level:

> **Day 1**: Firefighter circuit (HIIT cardiovascular capacity and strength training) and core strength training
> **Day 2**: Rest day
> **Day 3**: Upper-body (push/pull superset) strength training and flexibility
> **Day 4**: Rest day
> **Day 5**: Cardiovascular capacity (EBCT) and core strength training
> **Day 6**: Lower-body strength training and cardiovascular capacity training (HIIT)
> **Day 7**: Rest day

Each of these workouts should take approximately 45 to 60 minutes to complete.

Day 1: Firefighter Circuit (HIIT* & Strength Training) and Core			
Sequence	**Exercise**	**Reps/Duration**	**Rest Period**
Warm-Up	Jogging, Stationary Bike, Stair Climber, etc.	5 minutes	N/A
Firefighter Circuit** (3–4 Rounds)	Ground Ladder Lift, Carry, and Raise	50 feet	30 seconds
	Stair Climb	2 Stories, Up and Down for 30 seconds	30 seconds
	Tire/Dummy Drag (100–200 lbs.)	50 feet	30 seconds
	Battle Hose (50-foot OR 75-foot section of 1 3/4-inch or 2 1/2-inch)	30 seconds	30 seconds
	Ground Ladder Climb	Up and down for 30 seconds	30 seconds
Cool-Down	Walking, Jogging, Dynamic Stretching	5 minutes	N/A
Core Circuit (2 Rounds)	Standard or Elbow Plank	30–45 seconds	N/A
	Side Plank	30–45 seconds (both sides)	N/A
	Bridge Pose	30–45 seconds	N/A
	Hollow Rock	15–30 seconds	N/A
Flexibility Circuit (2 Rounds)	Downward Dog	30 seconds	N/A
	Child's Pose	30 seconds	N/A
	Runner's Lunge Stretch	30 seconds (Both Legs)	N/A
	Frog Pose	30 seconds	N/A
	Doorway Stretch for Chest	30 seconds	N/A
Foam Rolling	Legs, Hips, Back, Shoulders	5 minutes	N/A

**High-intensity interval training requires heart rate to be at or above 85 percent of maximum heart rate. If unable to monitor heart rate, push yourself to near-maximum exertion during the high-intensity intervals.

231

**For the firefighter circuit, consider the following stages of increasing difficulty:

Stage 1: Wear gym attire (shorts and t-shirt) only.

Stage 2: Add turnout coat and pants, boots, helmet, and gloves.

Stage 3: Add SCBA cylinder.

Stage 4: Add SCBA cylinder, SCBA mask on, and breathe air from cylinder.

At Level 2, execute the firefighter circuit starting at Stage 2 for two weeks, then Stage 3 for the next two weeks, and finally at Stage 4 for the final two weeks.

Day 2: Rest

Day 3: Upper-Body (Push/Pull Superset) Strength and Flexibility

Sequence	Exercise	Reps/Duration	Rest Period
Warm-Up	Jogging, Stationary Bike, Stair Climber, etc.	5 minutes	N/A
Upper-Body Circuit (3 Rounds)	Push-ups	AMRAP (As many reps as possible)	60 seconds
	Pull-ups	AMRAP	60 seconds
	Standing Chest Press with Cable Machine	10 reps	60 seconds
	Standing Cable Row	10 reps	60 seconds
	Medicine Ball Squat Press and Throw	10 reps	60 seconds
	Kneeling Cable Row (Hose Pulling or Hooking Ceiling Simulation)	10 reps (Both sides)	60 seconds

Sequence	Exercise	Reps/Duration	Rest Period
Flexibility/Yoga Circuit* (2 Rounds)	Downward Dog	30 seconds	N/A
	Baby Cobra Pose	30 seconds	N/A
	Pigeon Pose	30 seconds (both legs and hips)	N/A
	Child's Pose	30 seconds	N/A
	Garland Pose	30 seconds	N/A
	Modified Camel Pose	30 seconds	N/A
Foam Rolling	Upper body and back	5 minutes	N/A

*For an abundance of free yoga instructional videos and flexibility training routines, go to YouTube.com and search "beginner's or basic yoga for flexibility" or "flexibility training." There are also many gyms that offer basic yoga classes.

Day 4: Rest

Day 5: Cardiovascular Capacity (EBCT)* and Core Strength

Sequence	Exercise	Reps/Duration	Rest Period
Warm-Up	Jogging, Stationary Bike, Stair Climber, etc.	5 minutes	N/A
Medium of Your Choice* (Moderate Intensity)	Stair Climbing	30 minutes	N/A
	Swimming	30 minutes	N/A
	Cycling or Stationary Bike	30 minutes	N/A
	Running/Treadmill	30 minutes	N/A
	Rowing	30 minutes	N/A
	Elliptical Machine	30 minutes	N/A

233

Sequence	Exercise	Reps/Duration	Rest Period
Core Circuit (2 Rounds)	Crocodile Pose	30 seconds	N/A
	Child's Pose	30 seconds	N/A
	Side Plank	30–45 seconds (for both sides)	N/A
	Modified Superman	60 seconds (alternate holding sides for 10 seconds each)	N/A
	Hanging Leg Raise	AMRAP	N/A
	Weighted Side Bends	10 reps (both sides)	N/A
Cool-Down & Flexibility	Light Cardio Static Stretching	5–10 minutes	N/A
Foam Rolling	Legs and Hips	5 minutes	N/A

*Endurance-based cardiovascular training (EBCT) requires a heart rate at 70 to 85 percent of maximum heart rate. The exercise choices for EBCT can be broken down into shorter durations and mixed for a total of 30 to 60 minutes in one workout session. As long as one's heart rate stays in the 70 to 85 percent range, any exercise medium can be used for EBCT—traditional "cardio," strength training, yoga, etc. If unable to monitor heart rate, push yourself enough to elevate your respiratory rate moderately (but you should still be able to speak in full sentences).

Day 6: Lower-Body Strength and Cardiovascular Capacity (HIIT)

Sequence	Exercise	Reps/Duration	Rest Period
Warm-Up	Jogging, Stationary Bike, Stair Climber, etc.	5 minutes	N/A
Lower-Body Circuit (3 rounds)	Barbell Squats or Double Kettlebell Front Squats	10 reps	60 seconds
	Weighted Step-ups	10 reps (both legs)	60 seconds
	Barbell or Kettlebell Deadlifts	10 reps	60 seconds
	Walking Lunges (Weighted or Unweighted)	10 reps (both legs)	60 seconds
High-Intensity Interval Training Circuit (3 Rounds)	Battle Hose	30 seconds	30 seconds
	Stair or Hill Sprints	30 seconds	30 seconds
	Gym Mat Sled Push	30 seconds	30 seconds
	Firefighter Crawl	30 seconds	30 seconds
	Farmer's Carry With Heavy Equipment or Weight	30 seconds	30 seconds
Cool-Down	Walking, Jogging, Dynamic Stretching	5 minutes	N/A
Flexibility Circuit (2–3 Rounds)	Standing Hamstring Stretch	30 seconds	N/A
	Calf Stretch Against Wall (both legs)	30 seconds	N/A
	Runner's Lunge Stretch (both legs)	30 seconds	N/A
	Happy Baby Pose	30 seconds	N/A
	Pigeon Pose	30 seconds	N/A
Foam Rolling	Legs and Hips	5 minutes	N/A

Day 7: Rest

LEVEL 3: THE 5 TO 6-DAY WEEKLY PROGRAM

If the *Firefighter Functional Fitness Performance Assessment* placed you at *Level 3*, you will begin in the 5 to 6-day weekly program. Since you have been classified at the highest level of *Firefighter Functional Fitness*, this weekly program will challenge you to reach your optimal level of fireground performance:

> ▸ **Day 1**: Firefighter circuit (HIIT cardiovascular capacity and strength training) and core strength training
> ▸ **Day 2**: Lower-body and core strength training
> ▸ **Day 3**: Flexibility training
> ▸ **Day 4**: Cardiovascular capacity (EBCT) and Core strength training
> ▸ **Day 5**: Upper-body (push/pull superset) strength training
> ▸ **Day 6**: Optional: Choose from cardiovascular capacity (HIIT/EBCT), core, flexibility, or strength training.
> ▸ **Day 7**: Rest day

Each of these workouts should take approximately 45 to 60 minutes to complete.

Day 1: Firefighter Circuit (HIIT* & Strength Training and Core)			
Sequence	**Exercise**	**Reps/Duration**	**Rest Period**
Warm-Up	Jogging, Stationary Bike, Stair Climber, etc.	5 minutes	N/A
Firefighter Circuit** (4–5 Rounds)	Overhead Sledgehammer (Striking Tire)	10 reps with each arm leading, 30 second	15–30 seconds
	Stair Climb	2 Stories, up and down for 30 seconds	15–30 seconds
	Tire Drag (200 LBS.)	100 feet	15–30 seconds
	Firefighter Crawl	100 feet	15–30 seconds

Sequence	Exercise	Reps/Duration	Rest Period
	Farmer's Carry With Heavy Equipment (Saws or Extrication Tools)	100 feet	15–30 seconds
	Hose Hoist With Rope (50 foot Section OF 3-inch Hose Hoisted With Rope)	30 seconds	15–30 seconds
Cool-Down	Walking, Jogging, Dynamic Stretching	5 minutes	N/A
Flexibility Circuit (2–3 Rounds)	Supine Hamstring Stretch	30 seconds (both legs)	N/A
	Child's Pose	30 seconds	N/A
	Runner's Lunge Stretch	30 seconds (both legs)	N/A
	Butterfly Stretch	30 seconds	N/A
	Supine Figure 4 Stretch	30 seconds (both legs)	N/A
Foam Rolling	Legs, Hips, Back, Shoulders	5 minutes	N/A

*High-intensity interval training requires heart rate to be at or above 85 percent of maximum heart rate. If unable to monitor heart rate, push yourself to near-maximum exertion during the high-intensity intervals.

**For the firefighter circuit, consider the following stages of increasing difficulty:

Stage 1: Wear gym attire (shorts and t-shirt) only.

Stage 2: Add turnout coat and pants, boots, helmet, and gloves.

Stage 3: Add SCBA cylinder.

Stage 4: Add SCBA cylinder, SCBA mask on, and breathe air from cylinder.

At *Level 3*, we highly encourage functionally fit firefighters to complete firefighter circuits at either Stage 3 or 4.

Day 2: Lower-Body and Core Strength Training

Sequence	Exercise	Reps/Duration	Rest Period
Warm-Up	Jogging, Stationary Bike, Stair Climber, etc.	5 minutes	N/A
Lower-Body Circuit (4–5 Rounds)	Barbell Squats or Double Kettlebell Front Squats	10 reps	30–60 seconds
	Medicine Ball Squat Press and Throw	10 reps	30–60 seconds
	Barbell or Kettlebell Deadlifts	10 reps	30–60 seconds
	Lunges (Weighted or Unweighted)	10 reps (both legs)	30–60 seconds
Core Circuit (2–3 Rounds)	Supine Leg Lifts	10 reps	N/A
	Standard or Elbow Plank	60 seconds	N/A
	Cosmonaut Sit-Ups	10 reps	N/A
	Side Plank	60 seconds (both sides)	N/A
	Side Bend (Weighted or Unweighted)	10 reps (both sides)	N/A
Cool-Down	Light Cardio	5 minutes	N/A
Flexibility Circuit (2–3 Rounds)	Standing Hamstring Stretch	30 seconds	N/A
	Calf Stretch Against Wall (both legs)	30 seconds	N/A
	Runner's Lunge Stretch (both legs)	30 seconds	N/A
	Happy Baby Pose	30 seconds	N/A
	Pigeon Pose	30 seconds	N/A
Foam Rolling	Legs and Hips	5 minutes	N/A

Day 3: Flexibility Training			
Sequence	**Exercise**	**Reps/Duration**	**Rest Period**
Warm-Up	Jogging, Stationary Bike, Stair Climber, etc.	5 minutes	N/A
Flexibility/Yoga Circuit* (2–3 Rounds)	Child's Pose	30 seconds	N/A
	Downward Dog	30 seconds	N/A
	Baby Cobra Pose	30 seconds	N/A
	Cat Pose	30 seconds	N/A
	Pigeon Pose	30 seconds	N/A
	Happy Baby Pose	30 seconds	N/A
	Cow Pose	30 seconds	N/A
	Runner's Lunge Stretch	30 seconds (both legs)	N/A
	Standing or Supine Hamstring Stretch	30 seconds	N/A
	Chest Opener With Dowel Rod	10 reps	N/A
Foam Rolling	Total Body	5–10 minutes	N/A

*For an abundance of free yoga instructional videos and flexibility training routines, go to *YouTube.com* and search "beginner's or basic yoga for flexibility" or "flexibility training." There are also many gyms that offer basic yoga classes.

Day 4: Cardiovascular Capacity (EBCT)* and Core Strength			
Sequence	**Exercise**	**Reps/Duration**	**Rest Period**
Warm-Up	Jogging, Stationary Bike, Stair Climber, etc.	5 minutes	N/A
Medium of Your Choice* (Moderate Intensity)	Stair Climbing	30 minutes	N/A
	Swimming	30 minutes	N/A
	Cycling or Stationary Bike	30 minutes	N/A
	Running/Treadmill	30 minutes	N/A
	Rowing	30 minutes	N/A
	Elliptical Machine	30 minutes	N/A
Cool-Down	Light Cardio	5 minutes	N/A
Core Circuit (3 Rounds)	Plank (Standard or Elbow)	60 seconds	N/A
	Child's Pose	30 seconds	N/A
	Side Plank	60 seconds (both sides)	N/A
	Bridge Pose	60 seconds	N/A
	Hollow Rock	30–60 seconds	N/A
	Oblique Twist With Cable Machine or Elastic Band	10 reps (both sides)	N/A
Flexibility	Various Stretches	5 minutes	N/A
Foam Rolling	Legs and Hips	5 minutes	N/A

*Endurance-based cardiovascular training (EBCT) requires a heart rate at 70 to 85 percent of maximum heart rate. The exercise choices for EBCT can be broken down into shorter durations and mixed for a total of 30 to 60 minutes in one workout session. As long as one's heart rate stays in the 70 to 85 percent range, any exercise medium can be used for EBCT—traditional "cardio," strength training, yoga, etc. If unable to monitor heart rate, push yourself enough to elevate your respiratory rate moderately (but you should still be able to speak in full sentences).

Day 5: Upper-Body (Push/Pull Superset) Strength Training

Sequence	Exercise	Reps/Duration	Rest Period
Warm-Up	Jogging, Stationary Bike, Stair Climber, etc.	5 minutes	N/A
Upper-Body Circuit (4–5 Rounds)	Push-ups	AMRAP (as many reps as possible)	30–60 seconds
	Pull-ups	AMRAP	30–60 seconds
	Dips	AMRAP	30–60 seconds
	Inverted Rows	AMRAP	30–60 seconds
	Standing Overhead Press (Dumbbells or Kettlebells)	10 reps	30–60 seconds
	Angled Cable Row or Bent-Over Row	10 reps (both sides)	30–60 seconds
	Sled Push With Gym Mat (With or Without Weight on Mat)	50 feet	30–60 seconds
	Kneeling Cable Row (Hose Pulling or Hooking Ceiling Simulation)	10 reps (both sides)	30–60 seconds
Cool-Down	Static and Dynamic Stretching for Upper Body	5 minutes	N/A
Foam Rolling	Upper Body and Back	5 minutes	N/A

Day 6 (optional)

Your choice of the following: cardiovascular capacity (HIIT or ECBT), core, flexibility, or strength training. Get creative and blend two are more areas within one workout session.

Day 7: Rest

9 GUIDELINES TO SUCCESSFUL WORKOUT PROGRAMMING

As we wrap-up this chapter, we want to provide you with some guidelines for programming your weekly workouts.

1. **For the general population, 150 minutes of moderate-intensity exercise or 75 minutes of vigorous intensity exercise per week is recommended**. Due to firefighting's physical demands, *functionally fit firefighters will aim to double these weekly recommendations* primarily focusing on vigorous-intensity exercise.

2. **Cardiovascular capacity training can be performed as its own workout** (e.g. running, cycling, stair climbing, etc.). Functionally fit firefighters use both endurance-based cardiovascular training (heart rate at 70 percent of maximum heart rate) and high-intensity interval training (heart rate above 85 percent of maximum heart rate).

3. **Firefighting is a combination of cardiovascular capacity and muscular strength and endurance**. When possible, combine both of these elements into fitness circuits, complexes, HIIT, Tabata, etc. The ideal *Firefighter Functional Fitness* workout blends a firefighter wearing their PPE, specific firefighting tasks, cardiovascular capacity, and functional strength training.

4. **Core strength workouts can be incorporated into any workout, or they can be completed as stand-alone sessions**. When performing any movement or exercise, we should always focus on engaging our core. Our core is our center and it is where we harness the power to complete a multitude of tasks.

5. **Flexibility training should be incorporated into every workout session in some capacity**. Include flexibility training in warm-ups (dynamic stretching) and in cool-downs (static stretching). In addition, perform flexibility training as its own stand-alone workout as a 30 to 60-minute functional yoga or stretching session.

6. **Strength training should first focus on firefighter functional movements** (i.e. push, pull, lift, carry, and drag) **as opposed to targeting specific muscle groups** (e.g.

chest, biceps, abs). Functionally fit firefighters are primarily concerned with optimizing performance, not muscle growth.

7. **Allow 48 hours of rest for affected muscle(s) after strength training so that optimal recovery, repair, and rebuilding can occur**. Refer to *Pillar 2: Recovery and Rest* for more details on the four R's of strength training.

8. **As it pertains to strength training, adjust your loads, volumes, intensities and resting periods to suit your current level of strength**. For example, a deconditioned firefighter in *Level 1* will initially use lighter loads, volumes, and intensities (and longer rest periods) to progressively build muscular strength. Conversely, a well-conditioned firefighter in *Level 3* will be able to perform at greater capacity within each category because they have developed greater muscular strength.

9. **Every so often, take a week off**. There are both physical and mental benefits to this. It allows for a full body "reset" physically, and it keeps us from becoming either burned-out or bored of a particular regimen. There are varying opinions on how many weekly breaks should be taken in a year. At a minimum, strive for two to three breaks annually. During this time, continue flexibility and core training while you configure your next round of programming based on new goals that you set.

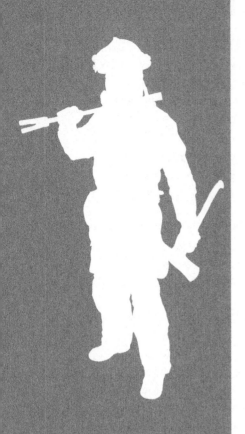

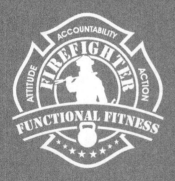

FIREFIGHTER
TOOLBOX

THE BIG 8 REVIEW

EXERCISES, STRETCHES, AND MOVEMENTS

For your convenience, here are the exercises, stretches, and movements introduced in the components of The Big 8.

By no means is this an exhaustive list of every exercise that you can use in your workouts. For example, there are more than 100 core strengthening exercises in existence; however, including all of them and their variations in one book would not be practical. Whatever you choose to include in your workouts, use the principles found in The Big 8 to guide you.

Visit FirefighterFunctionalFitness.com regularly for more workout programming ideas and functional fitness exercises, movements and stretches.

Core

> Plank (stand or forearm)
> Side plank (straight arm or forearm)
> Bridge Pose
> Side bends
> Standing oblique twist with elastic band or cable machine
> Modified Superman
> Downward Dog
> Supine Leg Raise
> Crocodile Pose
> Hollow Rock

Cardiovascular Capacity
Conventional High-Intensity Interval Training Exercises

> - Sprinting with jogging
> - Running stairs, step-mill, stair climber
> - Swimming
> - Stationary bike
> - Row machine
> - Boxing/punching bag
> - Jumping rope
> - Battle ropes
> - Plyometrics (box jumps, squat jumps, tuck jumps, etc.)
> - Strength training circuits (bodyweight exercises, dumbbell/weights, kettlebells, etc.)

Firefighter-Specific
High-Intensity Interval Training Exercises

> - Stair climber/ascending stairs
> - Jacobs Ladder
> - Ground ladder/aerial ladder climb
> - Ladder carry and raise
> - Firefighter Crawl
> - Forcible Entry Simulator
> - Sledgehammer tire strike
> - Heavy equipment carry
> - Battle Hose
> - Pulling ceiling simulation
> - Pulling charged hose line simulation
> - Equipment rope hoist
> - Hose Line Crawl
> - Hose Line Bear Crawl

Conventional Endurance-Based Cardiovascular Training Exercises

> Running
> Stationary bike, cycling, spinning
> Row machine
> Elliptical machine
> Swimming
> Walking stairs, step-mill, stair climber
> Group classes, exercise videos, boot camps

Flexibility

Back

> Child's Pose
> Cat Pose
> Cow Pose
> Two-knee twist

Core

> Modified Camel Pose
> Seated oblique twist
> Baby Cobra Pose
> Kneeling side stretch

Legs

> Supine hamstring stretch (against wall or with strap)
> Bent-over hamstring stretch
> Runner's lunge
> Downward Dog
> Calf stretch

Hip Complex

> Supine "Figure 4" stretch
> Seated "Figure 4" stretch
> Supine hip twist
> Pigeon Pose
> Dowel hip hinge

Groin

> Butterfly
> Frog Pose
> Supine groin and hip opener
> Garland Pose
> Happy Baby Pose

Chest

> Chest opener with dowel rod
> Hands together behind back
> Doorway stretch
> Parallel arm chest stretch

Neck

> Chin to chest
> Head to shoulder
> Lateral twist
> Chin pointed upwards

Arms and Shoulders

> Tricep stretch
> Medial arm stretch
> Wall stretches
> Arm circles
> Forearm stretch

The Push

> Push-ups
> Dips
> Standing overhead press
> Ground ladder lower and raise
> Medicine ball squat press and throw
> Squats
> Step-ups
> Sledgehammer strike
> Lunges
> Sled push with gym mat

The Pull

> Pull-ups
> Equipment Hoist
> Charged attack hose pull
> Single-arm angled cable row
> Double kettlebell swing
> Deltoid/reverse fly
> Battle hose
> Kneeling lateral cable row
> Bent-over row
> Inverted rows

The Lift

- Deadlifts
- Dumbbell scaptions
- Lunges
- Hose lifts for shoulder load carries
- Ladder lifts and carry variations
- Heavy tool lifts and carries
- Squats
- Upright row
- Patient lifts and transfers
- Plank variations

The Carry

- Farmer's carry
- Rack hold carry
- Overhead carry
- Shoulder carry (attack hose bundle)
- Over-the-shoulder carry (ladder)
- On-the-shoulder carry (ladder)
- Arms-length carry (ladder)
- Heavy tool carry
- Weighted lunges
- Hose carry on SCBA cylinder

The Drag

- Charged attack line drag—walking
- Charged attack line drag—kneeling
- Charged attack line drag—up stairs
- Supply line drag
- Downed firefighter drag
- Victim drag
- Tire drag
- Deadlifts
- Standing cable row
- Bear crawl and drag

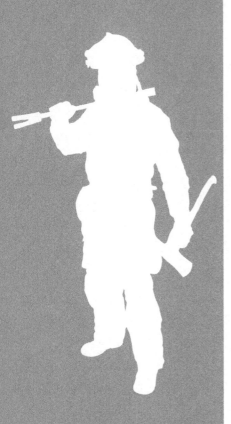

Success is no accident. It is hard work, perseverance, learning, studying, sacrifice, and most of all, love of what you are doing.

–PELÉ

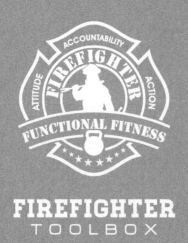

FIREFIGHTER
TOOLBOX

CHAPTER 17

ATTITUDE ACCOUNTABILITY ACTION

Anything worth having, anything worth achieving, must be earned. In firefighting, "taking the oath" puts you in rare company. But with this privilege comes tremendous responsibility—you must earn your spot every day in every way.

Functionally fit firefighters know the level of success they attain in the fire service will always be directly linked to their *attitude*, their level of personal *accountability*, and the ability to *act* upon their word. In order to become the best firefighter you can be, you must be more than the sum of your skills—you must be functionally fit, and you must *be* the example of firefighter fitness to those around you.

ATTITUDE

It is contagious.

We are affected by the attitudes of those around us, and our attitude has a tremendous effect on others as well. We have heard it many times: *Our attitude can make or break us.* In order to develop a proper attitude about our fitness, serious introspection is required.

> **❝❝ Functionally fit firefighters know that being fit for duty is a requirement of the job. Period."**

Think about this statement. What is your attitude about it? You must reflect on why you chose the path that you did. You must consider your level of commitment to the fire service, and as such, your commitment to personal health and fitness. The two are forever intertwined.

So ask yourself:

> ➤ What does my attitude say about me?
> ➤ Do I understand how many people depend on me?
> ➤ Do I show enthusiasm in taking care of myself?
> ➤ Do I demonstrate that there is more to the profession than just strategies, tactics, and skills?

Above all else, firefighter fitness requires a lifetime commitment that must be rooted in our own personal beliefs. If our attitude does not reflect the level of commitment the job demands, then we are already at a disadvantage.

In order to become the best firefighter you can be, you must be more than the sum of your skills—you must be functionally fit, and you must be the example of firefighter fitness to those around you.

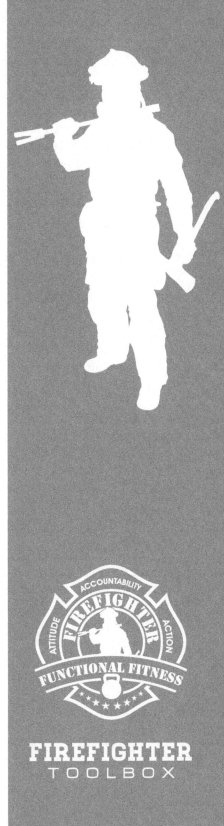

ACCOUNTABILITY

There are many opinions and definitions of personal accountability. To us, it simply means that *we own every decision we make*.

Perhaps one of the most important cornerstones of true personal accountability is that it is a full-time commitment—it is not something you can turn on and off as a matter of convenience. As a functionally fit firefighter, you must always hold yourself personally accountable if you are to be successful.

❝ Your fitness for duty is something that must be taken seriously. There are too many people that depend on you to take any other approach."

Are we suggesting perfection? *No*. Do we understand that there will be times when you will fall short and experience setbacks? *Yes, we all will*. However, a high level of personal accountability is what will carry you through the most difficult days, and it will push you even harder on your best days.

Put simply, your fitness for duty is something that must be taken seriously, because there are far too many people who depend on you: *Your family, fellow firefighters, and the public you serve*.

ACTION

❝ We all set an example. It takes courage, hard work, and commitment to set the right one for others to follow."

Clearly, none of what we have shared in this book means anything unless you *put it into action*. So, how can you achieve success with your functional fitness?

The 10 Commandments of
Firefighter Functional Fitness

1. **Use this book**. We have provided you with the tools and concepts needed to become a functionally fit firefighter. Use this book as a reference to establish and maintain your own personal functional fitness.

2. **Start small**. Small steps and incremental improvements will keep you from burning out. Functional fitness is more than simply "working out." It is a lifestyle comprised of many parts that when brought together, allows you to optimize your physical potential. By doing so, you will also benefit mentally and emotionally.

3. **Focus on your strengths**. Let them motivate you. Remember, your personal strengths are what got you this far. Don't ignore them. Use them to keep moving forward while you make an effort to improve on your weaknesses.

4. **Exercise when the timing is right**. Whenever you feel most motivated to exercise, that is when you should exercise. Some people enjoy working out in the morning, others may prefer the afternoon or evening. Whatever your preference, stick with it so it becomes part of your daily routine and lifestyle. Forcing yourself to work out when you're not "into it" may cause you to lose desire and consistency.

5. **Do something!** Remember that exercise and its benefits are cumulative, especially in strength training. If you can't make it to the gym, there are plenty of movements you can execute periodically throughout the day. For example, you could do 25 push-ups and 25 air squats several times throughout the day. By the end of the day, you could amass well over 200 reps for each exercise. Breaking up your exercise in this manner will also give you an energy boost and can help you mentally recharge, leading to better focus and productivity.

6. **Do what you like**. Some of us like to run, others do not. Some like to do yoga, others may not. Whatever you choose to incorporate into your fitness routine, make sure that it is effective, safe, and *functional for the job*.

7. **Show, don't just tell**. Let others see what you are doing. Be the one to set the right example through consistent exercise and healthy nutrition. Doing so will encourage positive peer pressure and spur others to join you on your fitness journey.

8. **Use the buddy system**. Find a workout partner to provide an extra level of accountability and commitment. Studies have shown that workout partners foster healthy competition, greater effort during exercise, and improved performance.

9. **Go the extra mile**. Ask your crewmates or others to work out with you while at the firehouse. They may decline your offer several times at first, but be persistent and open-minded.

10. **Share this book with other firefighters**. The information shared in this book is meant to be shared with your fellow firefighters. Remember: Their fitness level doesn't just impact them, it also impacts your safety and the community's safety.

A CALL TO ACTION

In this book, we have provided the knowledge, skills, and methods to help you optimize your functional fitness. But you must be the one to own and hone these principles to achieve personal success. *We gave you the tools, but you must do the work.*

Your dedication to *attitude, accountability,* and *action* will determine your level of success. Every day you will make the decision to own it because no one can do it for you. Adopting these principles will not only help you succeed, they will motivate those around you to succeed as well.

BONUS CHAPTERS

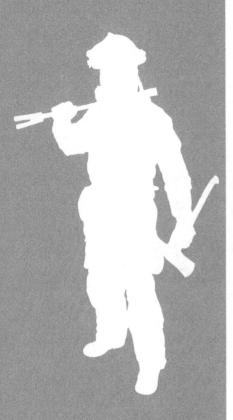

The number of health-related firefighter deaths suffered each year by the American fire service is simply unacceptable.

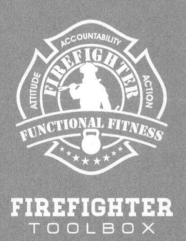

FIREFIGHTER
TOOLBOX

CHAPTER 18

THE IMPORTANCE OF ANNUAL MEDICAL EVALUATIONS

Every firefighter will agree the number of health-related LODDs the American fire service suffers each year is simply *unacceptable*. These LODDs are no more *a part of the job* than any other firefighter fatality. Yet, the leading causes of these deaths have remained constant: "stress and overexertion," mainly attributed to cardiovascular disease and heart attacks.

Functionally fit firefighters are champions of health and wellness. They understand medical evaluations are a critical, foundational component of their functional fitness. Medical evaluations are preventative, life-saving measures every firefighter and fire department should implement. However, like many other aspects of functional fitness, our medical evaluations *must be relevant to the tasks that we perform as firefighters*.

The National Fire Protection Association (NFPA) developed NFPA 1582 *Standard on Comprehensive Medical Program for Fire Departments* to document the specific recommended elements for firefighter medical evaluations. One of the most important aspects of this standard is it describes 13 essential firefighter job tasks that require us to maintain optimal physical and mental health. These job tasks are a common thread that have appeared throughout this book.

NFPA 1582 Highlights

➤ Wearing PPE and SCBA while performing firefighting tasks

➤ Exposure to toxic fumes

➤ Climbing flights of stairs while carrying equipment

➤ Being subjected to dehydration and elevated core temperatures

➤ Unpredictable emergency operations for extended periods of time requiring extreme exertion

➤ Ability to communicate effectively in high-stress environments while restricted by PPE and SCBA

➤ Critical, time-sensitive, and complex problem-solving during physical exertion in stressful and hazardous environments

This list is just a sample of the job tasks that regularly place tremendous physical and mental demands on our bodies and minds. In addition, we as human beings come "pre-packaged" with a variety of pre-existing medical conditions and family health histories that must also be considered. These physiological and hereditary factors increase our risk of acute health events when our bodies are forced to operate well beyond the range of normal cardiac and respiratory output.

In order to appropriately evaluate our ability to execute essential functions, it is necessary to move beyond the basic check-up that we receive from our family physicians. According to the International Association of Fire Chief's (IAFC) publication, *A Fire Department's Guide to Implementing NFPA 1582*, fire department physicians should24:

➤ Be a member of the department's Occupational Health and Safety Committee

➤ Understand demands placed on firefighters

➤ Understand the environmental working conditions of firefighters

➤ Use job descriptions provided by the department to determine a firefighter's medical clearance

Each and every firefighter in the American fire service is entitled to an annual occupational medical evaluation. It is incumbent upon fire service leadership to work through the barriers to implementing these examinations.

13 CRITICAL COMPONENTS TO FIREFIGHTER MEDICAL EVALUATIONS

While it is not the intent of this book to list each specific recommended requirement as indicated in NFPA 1582, the following is a list of medical evaluation components that every firefighter should have evaluated on an annual basis[25]:

> - Health risk appraisal
> - Work and medical history
> - Chest X-ray
> - Pulmonary function profile
> - Audiometric examination
> - Visual acuity with peripheral
> - Electrocardiogram (ECG) while resting
> - Blood pressure, height, weight, BMI
> - Colorectal stool screen
> - Complete lab analysis (blood and urine)
> - Hepatitis profile
> - Physical examination that includes cancer screening
> - Heavy metal exposure screening (as needed)

In addition to the examination elements, it is also recommended that a *fitness assessment* be conducted that includes:

> Body composition
> Sub-maximal VO$_2$ (cardiovascular capacity) treadmill test with 12-lead ECG
> Muscular strength (grip, arms, legs)
> Flexibility evaluation
> Individual report, counseling, and personalized exercise prescription

We will discuss firefighter fitness assessments in Chapter 21: *The Firefighter Physical Agility Assessment.*

COST VS. BENEFIT

One of the most common reasons for failure to implement annual medical evaluations is cost. In a study completed by the IAFC and the International Association of Firefighters (IAFF) and published in *A Fire Department's Guide to Implementing NFPA 1582,* control fire departments implementing an annual medical evaluation program averaged a 23 percent decrease in the cost per injury claim and a 28 percent decrease in days lost due to injury and illness as compared to pre-implementation data. The results also indicated a return on investment of approximately 1:2 (a return of approximately $2 for every $1 spent) after the first year of implementation. This figure also included start-up costs and capital expenditures. These numbers are conservative. They do not account for non-occupational injuries and increased medical costs which result from premature morbidity and mortality.

To assist departments seeking to implement annual medical evaluations, the IAFC Safety, Health, and Survival (SHS) Section authored the publication *A Fire Department's Guide to Implementing NFPA 1582.* You can download it in its entirety (free of charge) here:

https://www.iafc.org/files/1SAFEhealthSHS/shs_FDguideToImplementingNPFA1582.pdf

BECOME A CHAMPION OF HEALTH AND FITNESS

Functionally fit firefighters know that just as we cannot out-train a poor diet, we cannot expect a physical fitness regimen alone to prevent us from suffering a career-ending medical event or death. Annual medical evaluations are a vital and required aspect of comprehensive firefighter functional fitness. Not only can they identify otherwise unknown medical conditions but they also establish baseline medical data that is used to track a firefighter's health over the years. This can be critically important in the unfortunate event that a firefighter develops an occupational disease, because the records will support the need for crucial benefits covered under legislation (e.g. cancer presumption acts).

Firefighters who seek annual medical evaluations are true champions of firefighter health and fitness. Fire chiefs who require them for their firefighters are lifesavers. At the end of the day, those who benefit the most are our families, coworkers, and citizens.

ACTION STEPS:

1. Obtain a copy of NFPA 1582: Standard on Comprehensive Medical Programs for Fire Departments, and learn the components of a firefighter-specific annual medical evaluation.

2. Download and read A Fire Department's Guide to Implementing NFPA 1582, authored by Chief Jake Rhoades and Kim C. Favorite.

3. Establish a fitness and wellness committee in your fire department. Assign a member to identify local options available for administering NFPA 1582 compliant occupational medical assessments to all personnel.

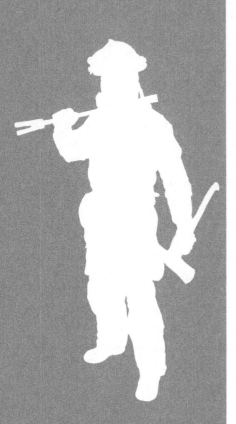

The shortest route to fewer firefighter deaths is through the heart.

—NATIONAL FALLEN FIREFIGHTERS FOUNDATION

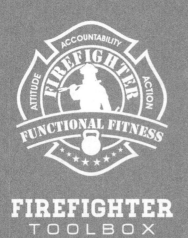

FIREFIGHTER
TOOLBOX

CHAPTER 19

WHAT IS KILLING FIREFIGHTERS? THE CARDIOVASCULAR EPIDEMIC

Although this book's primary goal is to help improve every firefighter's functional fitness, it also aims to mitigate one of the biggest issues within the fire service: health-related LODDs. We have discussed how to optimize firefighter performance. Additionally, we want firefighters to understand the gravity of the cardiovascular epidemic and the health dangers that we all face.

Our health and fitness is personal, but individual successes can and will have a tremendous impact on the fire service as a whole. This book is not intended to be the magic wand that will eliminate health-related LODDs. However, it is our goal to provide the tools and information every firefighter needs to help turn the tide. It is a comprehensive resource for you to use—not only to improve your own personal health but also to become a champion for firefighter health and fitness.

The fire service mission to serve others by saving lives and property comes with a

> **"When a firefighter dies in the line of duty, something went wrong."**
> -Dr. Burton Clark, EFO

whole host of risks that cannot be duplicated in any other profession. These risks drive us to seek constant improvement in our work in order to reduce the chance of injury and death. Yet, we also accept, as "part of the job," that we could die while carrying out our duties.

But there is a difference between *understanding* the risks associated with the job, and *accepting* them as a fact that we cannot change. Each year, the United States Fire Administration (USFA) compiles statistics that categorize firefighter LODDs. For several decades in the American fire service, we have acknowledged these statistics and worked to reduce the incidence of firefighter LODDs. Yet the numbers remain largely unchanged for more than 50 years.

So, what is killing firefighters?

Firefighters lose their lives for a variety of reasons. The USFA uses the following descriptions to categorize LODDs:

> - Stress and overexertion
> - Vehicle collisions
> - Lost or disoriented
> - Caught or trapped
> - Collapse
> - Struck by object
> - Fall
> - Other

No one can dispute the fact as firefighters we are at a much greater risk of injury and death than many other occupations. We do dangerous work, and we accept certain risks that are associated with this work. Historically, much of our focus in reducing LODDs has been in the area of fireground safety and other related categories. Yet, year after year, the category that stands out as the number one killer of firefighters is *stress and overexertion*.

Statistics at a Glance

Between 2005 and 2014, USFA statistics show *more than 50 percent* of the LODDs fell into the "stress and overexertion" category. This category is comprised of health-related deaths, which primarily include heart attack and stroke (see table 1). Although there was a dip in overall percentage in 2013, LODDs due to stress and overexertion in 2014 soared to 67 percent.

Table 19.1 – FIREFIGHTER LODDs CAUSED BY STRESS AND OVEREXERTION [26]			
Year	Number	Percent of Fatalities	Hometown Heroes
2014	61	67.0	22
2013	37	34.9	7
2012	45	55.5	13
2011	50	60.2	20
2010	55	63.2	16
2009	50	54.9	14
2008	54	45.0	12
2007	55	51.4	13
2006	55	53.9	15
2005	62	53.9	16

Source: United States Fire Administration.

No fire service professional can deny the fact our job requires us to be in top physical and mental shape. Everyone agrees that it is important, and everyone acknowledges that the LODD numbers are too high. However, putting actions to words is where we, as a profession, have failed on a national level.

> It is a significant fact that annually nearly half of all firefighter fatalities occur as a result of medical emergencies."
> —International Association of Fire Chiefs

Contrary to the views of some, *dying in the line-of-duty is not "part of the job."*

We do not pretend to believe that zero LODDs is immediately achievable, *but it should always be our goal.* We *can* have a tremendous impact on the things we can control, and the only way to realize a truly significant and lasting reduction in health-related LODDs is to take better care of ourselves. This starts with understanding the fire service's cardiovascular epidemic and knowing the specific cardiovascular stressors that every firefighter faces.

CARDIOVASCULAR DISEASE IN THE FIRE SERVICE

Cardiovascular disease (CVD) is made up of numerous separate disease processes that adversely affect the heart and blood vessels. If a firefighter has CVD, they face an increased risk of cardiovascular events, which include heart attack, heart arrhythmias, heart valve problems, stroke, and more.

CVD is the leading cause of firefighter LODDs. It is attributed to approximately half of on-duty firefighter fatalities. *Coronary heart disease* (CHD) is the primary culprit, causing 45 percent of all firefighter LODDs. By comparison, LODDs from CHD for law enforcement and emergency medical services are at 22 percent and 11 percent, respectively[27].

> " When combined with a firefighter's extreme physical workload and hot environment, the risk of a sudden cardiac event or death increases 136 times during firefighting activities."
>
> -Dr. Stefanos Kales

Why is this figure so much higher for firefighters?

For every firefighter LODD due to CVD, there are roughly 25 nonfatal cardiac events. Annually, this translates to roughly 850 on-duty, nonfatal cardiac events (i.e. heart attacks, strokes, arrhythmias, etc.) for firefighters. Additionally, the probability of a sudden cardiac event or death is more than 100 times greater during fire suppression duties as compared to nonemergency duties. Having a major heart attack or stroke is debilitating and usually career-ending for firefighters.

What Are the Cardiovascular Disease Risk Factors for Firefighters?

Risk factors for a cardiovascular event are broken down into two categories: *non-modifiable* and *modifiable*.

Non-modifiable risk factors cannot be changed. These include age, gender, and inherited and genetic conditions. Simply put, these are the risk factors that we are born with. Unfortunately, some of us are dealt an unfair hand in the game of "genetics poker." The cards we are dealt may include an elevated risk of cardiovascular disease (e.g. high cholesterol, congenital heart disease, blood clotting disorders, etc.). Just like the inherent risks of the fireground, we cannot completely control or eliminate non-modifiable risk factors; however, we can significantly manage them through *Firefighter Functional Fitness*' comprehensive approach.

Modifiable risk factors can be improved to lessen the risk of CVD. These include physical activity, exercise, nutrition, tobacco use, high blood pressure, high cholesterol, obesity, diabetes, and certain occupational factors. Within this book, we have focused on reducing modifiable risk factors, specifically through improving our physical activity, exercise, and nutrition.

Unfortunately, the list of modifiable risk factors is long for firefighters. All of the following increase our risk of experiencing a CVD-related event[28]:

> Sedentary lifestyle
> Poor nutrition
> Tobacco use (including smokeless tobacco)
> Sleep deprivation
> Noise (station tones, alerts, environmental)
> Obesity
> Diabetes
> Hypertension (high blood pressure)
> High cholesterol
> Exposure and inhalation of smoke gases and particulates (acute and chronic)
> Physically-demanding firefighting duties
> Sympathetic nervous system activation
> Environmental or thermal stress
> Dehydration
> Post-traumatic stress disorder

Table 19.2 – HEART DISEASE AND FIREFIGHTER SUDDEN CARDIAC DEATH	
Prior diagnosis of heart disease	35 times greater odds
Older than 45 years old	18 times greater odds
Hypertension	12 times greater odds
Diabetes	10.2 times greater odds
Smoking tobacco	8.6 times greater odds
High cholesterol	4.4 times greater odds
Obesity	3.1 times greater odds

We will discuss several of these cardiovascular disease catalysts and explain how they can negatively affect firefighters.

Hypertension

Hypertension, also known as *high blood pressure*, is a serious problem in the fire service. It is estimated that 20 to 30 percent of all firefighters have hypertension. In a study of firefighters with hypertension, 75 percent were lacking appropriate medical treatment[29].

Uncontrolled hypertension can be extremely dangerous for firefighters. It causes stiffening of blood vessels and an increased risk of CHD, stroke, and kidney disease. Hypertension also leads to left ventricular hypertrophy (heart enlargement which causes it to work harder while pumping blood). Of the firefighter LODDs due to CHD, 56 percent were found to have left ventricular hypertrophy, most likely due to hypertension.

> ❝ If a firefighter has hypertension, they are 12 times more likely to suffer sudden cardiac death while performing firefighting duties.”

WHAT IS KILLING FIREFIGHTERS? THE CARDIOVASCULAR EPIDEMIC

Diabetes

Diabetes is the elevated blood glucose ("blood sugar") concentration due to insulin deficiency or insulin resistance. Unfortunately, those who have diabetes also tend to have hypertension and high cholesterol—both of which are risk factors for CHD. As it pertains to line-of-duty heart disease events and retirements, diabetes was present in 21 percent and 26 percent, respectively[30].

> ❝ If a firefighter has diabetes, they are 10.2 times more likely to suffer sudden cardiac death while performing firefighting duties."

Obesity

Obesity is a primary gateway to hypertension, high cholesterol, diabetes, stroke, CHD, sleep apnea, liver and gallbladder disease, cancer, dementia, and more. In a recent study, the National Volunteer Fire Council reports approximately 77 percent *of the American fire service is overweight*. Unfortunately, this figure directly reflects the obesity epidemic of the American population.

Technically speaking, obesity is characterized as having a body mass index (BMI) of greater than 30 kg/m^2 or a total body fat of greater than 25 percent of one's total body weight. In the 1980s, the average veteran firefighter's BMI was 26 kg/m^2. By the year 2001, it had increased to 29.7 kg/m^2. Regrettably, the incidence and severity of obesity continues to increase year after year in the fire service[31].

> ❝ If a firefighter has obesity, they are 3.1 times more likely to suffer sudden cardiac death while performing firefighting duties."

High Cholesterol

Due to the nature of our profession, we have very erratic eating habits. Eating meals at irregular times leads us to choose foods that are the most convenient. Many of these "foods of convenience" are overly-processed, and have high amounts of trans fats, refined carbohydrates, sugars, and sodium (e.g. fast food, pizza, cheeseburgers, etc.). These are the same foods that directly increase the risk of heart disease by detrimentally altering HDL/LDL cholesterol ratios.

> ❝ If a firefighter has high cholesterol, they are 4.4 times more likely to suffer sudden cardiac death while performing firefighting duties."

Tobacco Use

Tobacco products negatively affect blood pressure, cholesterol, and carbon monoxide levels in our bodies. Smoking increases the risk of heart attack by increasing platelet aggregation (i.e. stickiness), damaging blood vessel linings, and decreasing coronary blood and oxygen flow.

> ❝ Cigarette smokers face a two to fourfold increased risk of developing heart disease."

Cigarette smokers face a two to fourfold increased risk of developing heart disease. Secondhand smoke increases a nonsmoker's risk of developing CHD by 25 to 30 percent. Smokers die an average of 13.8 years earlier than non-smokers[32].

For firefighters who succumbed to CVD-related LODDs, an astonishing 40 to 50 percent were smokers[33]. Smokeless tobacco is less harmful than its counterpart, but its users also face an increased risk of heart attack, stroke, and throat and mouth cancer.

The *Firefighter Functional Fitness* philosophy always aims to achieve balance and moderation for our fitness and nutrition. Tobacco use, however, does not fit into this philosophy. *It should be avoided at all costs*. If you don't currently use tobacco products, continue on this path. If you use tobacco, the best time to quit is *now*. If you currently smoke cigarettes and have considered quitting, know this: After a year of being smoke-free, your risk of heart disease is cut in half [34].

For chiefs and firefighters, we encourage you to not only fight for a tobacco-free workplace, but to also to implement a strict tobacco-free policy at your fire department. This may mean incentivizing current firefighters who smoke to quit. For new applicants and newly-hired firefighters, make it clear that being tobacco-free is a condition of their employment or membership.

> ❝ If a firefighter smokes tobacco, they are 8.6 times more likely to suffer sudden cardiac death while performing firefighting duties."

Psychological Stress

Stress from the fire scene, the firehouse, and home all cause detrimental effects on our bodies. Stress elevates our heart rate, blood pressure, cholesterol, leads to poor sleeping habits, and CVD. Due to the intense and sometimes horrific circumstances of our incidents, firefighters may develop post-traumatic stress disorder (PTSD). Unfortunately, PTSD and PTSD-related suicide are also on the rise in the fire service.

If you are a firefighter who is suffering from psychological, mental or emotional stress, depression, or thoughts of suicide, don't be afraid to reach out to get help. Contact any of the following resources for help:

> ▸ **Firefighter Behavioral Health Alliance**:
>   847-209-8208, ffbha.org
> ▸ **National Volunteer Fire Council's Share the Load Program**:
>   888-731-3473, nvfc.org
> ▸ **Station House Retreat**:
>   855-525-4357, StationHouseRetreat.com

Sleep Deprivation

Firefighting is not a Monday through Friday, "9 to 5" job. Firefighters, especially volunteer firefighters, are almost always on call—day and night, 365 days per year. Therefore, nighttime calls disrupt our sleep patterns and cause sleep deprivation.

Chronic sleep deprivation leads to altered diet, physical inactivity, psychological stress, disrupted circadian rhythms, and metabolic changes—all of which contribute to obesity, diabetes, hypertension, and CVD.

Read more on how sleep deprivation affects our well-being and get tips to optimizing your sleep in *Pillar 2: Recovery and Rest.*

THE CARDIOVASCULAR EFFECTS OF SMOKE EXPOSURE

We have long known that firefighting smoke and vehicle exhaust contain numerous carcinogens. However, much of the fire service does not yet understand many of these toxins also play a serious role in heart attack, stroke, and CVD.

Here is *just a fraction* of the hundreds of toxins and irritants found in the smoke that firefighters are exposed to[35]:

> ‣ Acetaldehyde
> ‣ Acrolein
> ‣ Benzene
> ‣ Carbon monoxide
> ‣ Formaldehyde
> ‣ Glutaraldehyde
> ‣ Hydrogen cyanide
> ‣ Hydrogen chloride
> ‣ Hydrogen sulfide
> ‣ Nitrogen dioxide
> ‣ Phosgene

> ➤ Respirable dust, fiberglass, and other airborne particles
> ➤ Styrene
> ➤ Sulfur dioxide

The major chemical asphyxiants in smoke, *carbon monoxide* and *hydrogen cyanide*, impede cellular oxygenation and transport within the body. Carbon monoxide binds to hemoglobin, preventing oxygen from being carried to the necessary tissues. Hydrogen cyanide renders cells useless through anaerobic metabolism and lactic acidosis.

These two processes are of particular importance to a firefighter's cardiovascular and respiratory systems since both are already working at or beyond maximum physical capacity. With increased metabolic and oxygen demands, carbon monoxide and hydrogen cyanide reduce cardiovascular capacity. Therefore, they increase a firefighter's acute risk for heart attack and stroke. These toxins also accelerate the long-term development of atherosclerosis (i.e. development of fatty deposits, plaque, and narrowing of the arteries). Atherosclerosis is a major component of CVD, which also predisposes firefighters to heart attack and stroke.

THE CARDIOVASCULAR STRAIN OF FIREFIGHTING

There are numerous ways that firefighting duties detrimentally affect our cardiovascular system. As it pertains to acute cardiovascular strain (i.e. cardiac workload), there are four primary culprits: *sympathetic nervous system activation*, *physical exertion*, *environmental or heat stress*, and *dehydration*. Let's examine how each affect our bodies during firefighting activities.

Sympathetic Nervous System Activation

Within our bodies, the sympathetic nervous system releases endorphins (i.e. epinephrine and cortisol) as a response to stressful stimuli. These endorphins rapidly increase heart rate and sustain it for prolonged periods of time. Studies have shown that the audible alert and instantaneous light from a station's dispatch will increase

275

a firefighter's heart rate to maximum or near-maximum capacity within a matter of seconds. These studies also demonstrated that endorphins cause firefighters' heart rates to stay elevated for approximately three hours *after* a strenuous alarm response[36].

An elevated, sustained heart rate causes increased *cardiac workload* and *oxygen consumption*—two factors that put incredible strain on the heart. Functionally fit firefighters with *optimal cardiovascular capacity* have been proven to demonstrate significantly lower heart rates during pre- and post-alarm times—as compared to firefighters who solely focus on strength training[37]. Improving your cardiovascular capacity through frequent exercise decreases the cardiac strain that your heart experiences during and after an alarm response.

Physical Exertion

To say that firefighting is a "physical job" is truly an understatement. The strenuous workload of firefighting comes from advancing hose lines, carrying heavy tools and equipment, forcing entry, carrying and climbing ladders, rescuing victims, etc. Firefighters complete all of the tasks while wearing personal protective equipment that adds weight, restricts movement, increases heart rate, reduces cardiovascular capacity, inhibits body heat release, and reduces physical performance.

The actual oxygen consumption rate of firefighting activities has been measured and quantified. These activities carry identical metabolic and oxygen requirements of professional athletes. Any cardiovascular deficiency that a firefighter may have will be exposed and magnified on the fireground, where firefighters frequently exceed their theoretical maximum heart rates. As we have witnessed year after year, such cardiovascular strain has proven to be lethal to a firefighter's heart.

Environmental and Heat Stress

There a several factors that cause environmental (heat) stress for firefighters: personal protective equipment (PPE), the fire environment, and metabolic activities. PPE is insulated with multiple layers, and these layers severely limit body heat release. The fire environment itself ranges from ambient temperatures to more than 500 degrees Fahrenheit. Additionally, firefighting duties cause our core body temperature to increase. All of these factors increase heart rate and multiply cardiovascular strain.

> " Probably the greatest stress ever imposed on the human cardiovascular system is the combination of exercise and hyperthermia. Together these stresses can present life-threatening challenges, especially in highly-motivated athletes who drive themselves to extremes in hot environments."
> —L.B. Rowell, In Human Cardiovascular Physiology

Dehydration

Due to physical exertion and environmental stress, firefighters can sweat out almost 2 liters per hour while on the fireground. Dehydration leads to serious cardiovascular strain for multiple reasons: 1) it decreases blood plasma volume, 2) it decreases cardiac output, and 3) it increases the formation of blood clots. These three processes are all predisposing factors to heart attack and stroke. To read more about how dehydration affects firefighters, please read *Pillar 3: Hydration*.

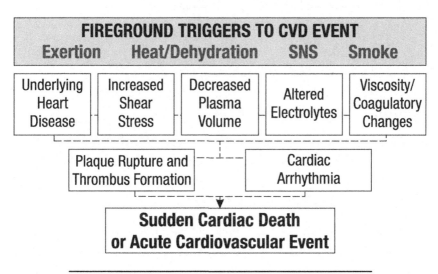

Source: Denise L. Smith, David A. Barr, and Stefanos N. Kales

---

* Smith, D. L., Barr, D. A., & Kales, S. N. (2013). Extreme sacrifice: Sudden cardiac death in the U.S. fire service. *Extreme Physioogy and Medicine*, Retrieved from http://extremephysiolmed.biomedcentral.com/articles/10.1186/2046-7648-2-6

CONCLUSION: KNOW THY ENEMY

In working towards eliminating the cardiovascular epidemic in the fire service, we must define and examine the problem to know what we are up against. The modifiable and non-modifiable risk factors that firefighters face must be hit head-on if we are going to truly reduce health-related LODDs.

The information presented in this chapter is not meant to scare firefighters. Rather, it illustrates the daunting, yet realistic challenges we face in our profession. As functionally fit firefighters, we must use this information as motivation to make our fitness and health the top priorities.

Now is the time to change the way we approach our own health. We cannot simply acknowledge the facts; we must also work to change our mentality and behavior. Ignoring and neglecting firefighter fitness is no longer an option. We can no longer accept the complacency and apathy that have long plagued the fire service. If we are to change the tide, we must be champions of firefighter fitness on a personal and professional level.

Special Acknowledgement

Thank you to the International Association of Firefighters, Dr. Stefanos N. Kales, and Dr. Albert Rielly for producing the document: *Heart Disease in the Fire Service*. If it was not for their efforts, this chapter would not have been possible.

To read the full document, please visit: https://www.iaff.org/hs/PDF/HeartDiseaseManual_2013.pdf

ACTION STEPS:

1. Control what you can control. Manage your modifiable risk factors by participating in 150 minutes of vigorous exercise every week. In addition to frequent exercise, balance recovery, hydration, and proper nutrition.

2. If you use tobacco, quit as soon as possible. If the use of tobacco products is still permitted at your fire department, fight for a tobacco-free workplace.

3. Minimize your cancer and cardiovascular risks by following these guidelines:

   - Commit to "wearing your air" during fire extinguishment, smoke exposure, and during overhaul.

   - Perform gross decontamination of your PPE while on scene.

   - Use body wipes to clean vascular areas of your skin (i.e. head, neck, armpits, hands, groin etc.) after smoke exposure.

   - Back at the firehouse, launder your PPE (e.g. coat, pants, hood, gloves) in an extraction washer. Then launder your uniforms and clothing as soon as possible.

   - Shower immediately with a degreasing soap.

4. Whether you are a chief or a rookie firefighter, your personal example of fitness will speak volumes to other firefighters. Ask fellow firefighters to workout with you and eat healthy meals with you.

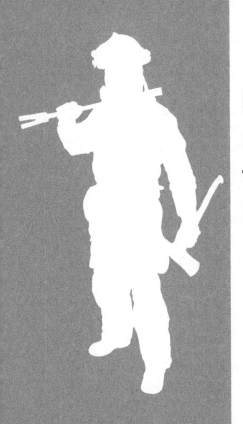

Regardless of rank, we are all firefighters at heart.

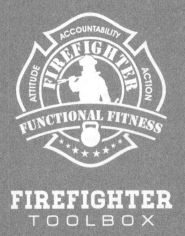

FIREFIGHTER
TOOLBOX

CHAPTER 20

FOR THE FIRE CHIEF: OVERCOMING ORGANIZATION BARRIERS TO FIREFIGHTER FITNESS

Up to this point, we have focused on how *individual firefighters* can improve their functional fitness. We will now shift gears and discuss how you, the fire chief, can make fitness and health a priority for the firefighters in your organization.

Regardless of rank, we are all firefighters at heart. As such, we can easily agree our levels of health and fitness are directly linked to our fireground performance. We know they can have a tremendous impact on the opportunity for a long and healthy career and retirement. Yet across the country, fire departments struggle with the implementation of fitness programs designed to take care of their own, even in the face of undeniable statistics that prove health-related LODDs are our number one killer.

In the fire service, there is a set of obligations we can all agree on regardless of paid or volunteer status, whether an organization has 1 station or 100. Core values such as *service, dedication, humility,* and the *duty* to save lives and protect property are innate in our profession. Yet the very idea of implementing firefighter fitness programs is often viewed differently from organization to organization, and these viewpoints result in a range of real and perceived barriers.

Why is this? Are there really that may barriers?

Over the years, numerous studies have focused on the challenges of implementing firefighter fitness programs. While it is certainly not a one-dimensional issue, the barriers can be more specific than we might realize. While it would be pretentious of us to tell you that we have all the answers to this dilemma, we will offer some solutions to overcoming organizational barriers to firefighter health and fitness.

HOW TO OVERCOME BARRIERS TO FIREFIGHTER FITNESS: PERCEPTION VS. REALITY

1. Determine the Problem

In life and in the fire service, failure to correct problems is often a result of being reactionary. We all agree on the importance of being fit for duty, but narrowly focused attempts to address firefighter fitness problems are often made at the organizational level to correct a problem that is more complex than we might realize. For example: A fire department that attempts to improve firefighter fitness levels by providing gym memberships to its members *without* formal policy, enforcement, guidance, and data collection will have fewer chances of success than a department that implements a program that has been researched, vetted, and agreed upon by all parties involved.

What you think you know and how it should be handled can be quite different than what the facts demonstrate. Addressing and improving firefighter fitness at an organizational level is not something that can be done in a vacuum. As the fire chief, your first step in moving toward a solution to the problem is to learn where the barriers exist in your department and whether they are workforce concerns, management concerns, or both.

The bottom line: Within your organization, you must first discover and understand the root cause of the barriers if you are going to create realistic and successful solutions. Organizational barriers can exist in several areas. They include:

> Departmental social norms and culture
> Work rules and obligations
> Management support and style

2. Departmental Social Norms and Culture: Polling

First and foremost, you must understand and accept there are many aspects of fire department culture that are good. All too often, the word "culture" carries a negative connotation in the fire service. It can easily polarize us if we are not careful, as has been seen time and time again on a number of issues that strike emotional chords with firefighters. So, you must ask yourself: *How do you protect the successful aspects of your organization's fire service culture while infusing improvements that are sorely needed at the same time?* In other words, how do you keep what works and improve what does not?

One of the easiest ways to learn more about what barriers to firefighter fitness

> **" Firefighter fitness is about attitude, accountability, and action. Fire chiefs must do a better job of promoting a culture of fitness and leading by example."**

exist in your organization is simply to ask your members. Polling the "rank and file" with a well-developed questionnaire can provide valuable insight into how the organization's culture and social norms affect attitudes about firefighter fitness. Moreover, it is likely that you will also find clues about what might increase support for firefighter fitness programs.

Will you ever get 100 percent buy-in? Probably not. Remember: Even if an organization's culture seems to be a deterrent to implementing change, fitness is still personal. But including your most important assets (your people) in solutions to problems will prove very beneficial in the end, as long as you are willing to listen to them. As a leader, you must be willing to listen, and you must also be willing to make people feel uncomfortable from time to time as a catalyst for improvement.

3. Work Rules and Obligations: Fact-Finding and Assigning Responsibility

A **united** approach to overcoming firefighter fitness barriers will often produce tangible results. While there may be conflict in the initial stages, a properly formed committee that includes management and labor, as well as subject matter experts in fitness, nutrition, insurance, and worker's compensation can quickly sort through the myths associated with firefighter fitness. Even more importantly, a working committee can assign action items to each member.

Consider researching previously published applied research projects and dissertations on the subject matter. Firefighter fitness is a widely researched subject area. From clinical studies to applied research projects, there are many departments and organizations across the country that have not only done the research but have implemented programs as a result.

We have said it before, and we will say it again: *Talk is cheap. Actions speak louder than words.* Infusing improvements into an existing culture requires **action**.

Obstacles and myths that can be overcome in fact-finding include:

> - Cost vs. benefit (return on investment)
> - Program responsibility
> - Funding options
> - In-house trainers vs. external certified personal trainers and programs
> - Fitness policy creation and the approval process
> - Legal concerns and insurance considerations

4. Management Support and Style

At the end of the day, it is your leadership and administration that will make or break your organization's fitness program. As the fire chief, *you must be honest with yourself.* Where do you stand on the issue? Are you stuck in an intellectual agreement that lacks action? Or do you personally promote "white shirt fitness" by frequently engaging in exercise?

> " Part of leading by example is recognizing that, as chiefs, we are not exempt from the 'shalls.'"
> -Jake Rhoades, Fire Chief, Kingman Fire Department, Arizona

Above all else, the most powerful influence you have is demonstrating your personal commitment to firefighter fitness thorough your own actions. Make sure that your firefighters see you working out on a regular basis. Encourage them to exercise with you. As your schedule permits, cook and eat healthy meals with them.

A key factor in the overall success of firefighter fitness programs is the level of support and enthusiasm that an administration has for their members' fitness. Without communication of organizational expectations (and action-oriented support from management), firefighters are left to deal with fitness for duty on their own. The resulting lack of direction and perceived lack of support spells failure in most cases, except for the most self-motivated firefighters.

Management must take the initiative. Demonstrate a high level of concern for your organization's people by appointing a health and safety officer who is not only qualified to administer a fitness program but is also enthusiastic about it. Communicate the benefits of firefighter fitness and educate personnel on the potential harmful effects of poor personal fitness. Phasing in a fitness program that has been vetted by a committee of stakeholders and that includes key components (as outlined in NFPA 1583) is a good place to start.

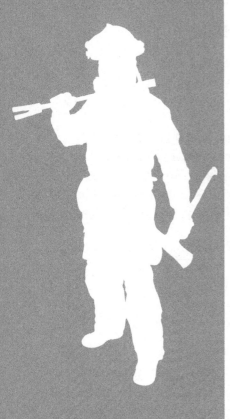

Providing professional guidance, allowing personnel to work out on-duty, then moving toward a requirement for exercise and periodic physical agility assessments are all ingredients in the recipe for long-term firefighter fitness success.

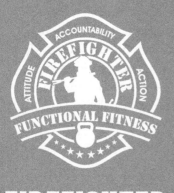

FIREFIGHTER
TOOLBOX

WHAT SUCCESS LOOKS LIKE

The success of any fitness program depends on a number of variables. First and foremost, management support and cooperation with workforce representatives is required. Management must be an active participant, both administratively and functionally. Fire department administrators must solicit appropriate guidance, consider the use of trained professionals, employ positive peer pressure from the bottom up and the top down, and develop policies that enforce a positive, non-punitive approach to fitness.

There is no requirement that a fire chief or line officer has to be the one in charge of implementing a fitness program. Regardless of rank, we all must be champions of fitness, fully willing to promote it and motivate others to be the best they can be. Every firefighter must be able to count on the support of their administration through policy implementation, peer support, and, most importantly, actions that demonstrate a willingness to be a part of the solution.

ACTION STEPS:

1. If you aren't currently participating in a regular fitness regimen, get started as soon as possible. Set an example for firefighters under your command.

2. As a fire chief, it is critical that you read, know, and implement NFPA 1583: *Standard on Health-Related Fitness Programs for Fire Department Members*.

3. For further reading on implementing a successful fitness program at your organization, please read Dan Kerrigan's *Identifying Fitness Strategies for the East Whiteland Fire Department*: http://www.nfa.usfa.fema.gov/pdf/efop/efo47062.pdf

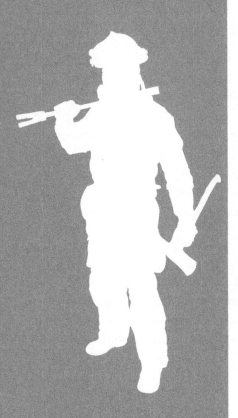

Citizens expect the highest level of service and physical performance from their firefighters. No exceptions.

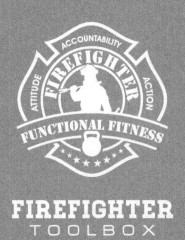

ACCOUNTABILITY
ATTITUDE
FIREFIGHTER
ACTION
FUNCTIONAL FITNESS

FIREFIGHTER
TOOLBOX

CHAPTER 21

THE FIREFIGHTER PHYSICAL AGILITY ASSESSMENT

We shared methods and tools to help maximize firefighter functional fitness, health, and wellness. We also discussed the importance of fire departments providing annual medical evaluations for their firefighters. In addition to medical evaluations, a comprehensive fitness and wellness program should incorporate periodic fitness assessments to ensure that firefighters remain *fit for duty* throughout the entirety of their careers.

In this chapter, we will discuss the need for fire departments to require annual firefighter physical agility assessments (PAA), and we will provide guidance on how to implement a PAA at your fire department.

WHAT IS A PHYSICAL AGILITY ASSESSMENT?

In its most basic form, a PAA is simply a firefighter functional fitness test. Its purpose is to assess a firefighter's muscular strength, endurance, and power; cardiovascular capacity; and ability to perform realistic fireground functions. During a PAA, firefighters perform 5 to 10 firefighting tasks to simulate the physical demands of the fireground. As a functionally fit firefighter, you will have no difficulty completing this assessment. More than anything, it should serve as validation for all of your functional fitness training.

WHY IS A PHYSICAL AGILITY ASSESSMENT NECESSARY?

As recruits in the fire academy, most firefighters participate in a PAA as a requirement for entry and/or graduation. Additionally, when candidates seek employment at prospective fire departments, it is customary that the hiring process involves some form of PAA or CPAT (Candidate Physical Abilities Test).

> " Firefighters gain an average of 2.2 pounds a year."
> -Dr. Sara A. Jahnke

Unfortunately, after firefighters get hired and are "on the job," many departments do not require periodic fitness evaluations or testing to ensure their firefighters can satisfactorily perform physical job functions.

We are often asked by members of the public if fire departments require annual fitness tests for firefighters. Our response of "*many do not*" leaves the civilians in a state of disbelief. This is because all citizens expect the highest level of service and physical performance from their firefighters. Instituting an annual PAA is a form of accountability. It determines a firefighter's level of functional fitness and physical performance.

HOW TO CREATE A PHYSICAL AGILITY ASSESSMENT

Creating a firefighter PAA is easier than most might think. It should possess some combination of the following firefighting tasks to gauge a firefighter's performance:

> ‣ Pulling supply hose
> ‣ Stretching uncharged attack hose
> ‣ Pulling, dragging, and crawling with charged attack hose
> ‣ Connecting supply hose to a hydrant
> ‣ Carrying, raising, and climbing ground ladders
> ‣ Forcible entry simulation (e.g. door simulator or Keiser Force™ Machine)

> Vertical (roof) ventilation simulation
> Lifting, carrying, and hoisting firefighting equipment
> Ascending stairs with firefighting equipment
> Dragging a victim to safety

While completing the PAA, the firefighter should wear their normally assigned turnout gear, including a helmet, boots, gloves, and SCBA. The goal is to make the physical demands of the assessment directly reflect those of the fireground. It is each agency's decision as to whether or not the firefighter should perform none, some, or all of the PAA while breathing from their SCBA.

Each fire department should create a PAA that most closely represents their typical fireground functions. The following example is the PAA from the Metro West Fire Protection District of St. Louis County, Missouri.

Station 1: Supply Hose Carry and Hydrant Connection

The firefighter will pull and drag 5-inch supply hose a total of 50 feet to a hydrant. The firefighter will then remove the large diameter discharge cap and connect the supply hose to the hydrant. The firefighter will walk 50 feet to the next station.

Station 2: Uncharged Attack Hose Line Advancement

The firefighter will pull and drag an uncharged 1 3/4-inch attack hose 150 feet and drop the hose to the ground. The firefighter will walk 150 feet to the next station.

Station 3: Ground Ladder Carry and Raise

The firefighter will pull a 14-foot roof ladder from the ladder bed of a fire truck and carry it 50 feet to a nearby building, where the firefighter will raise it to the second story windowsill. The firefighter will walk 50 feet to the next station.

Station 4: Ladder Climb

The firefighter will climb a prepositioned ground ladder and touch the second story windowsill. The firefighter will descend the ladder and will walk 25 feet to the next station.

Station 5: Forcible Entry Simulation

Using the Keiser Force™ Machine, the firefighter will strike and drive a weighted metal sled 60 inches. The firefighter will walk 10 feet to the next station.

Station 6: Mask Up and Hose Bundle Carry

The firefighter will don their SCBA mask and breathe from their SCBA cylinder for the remainder of the PAA. The firefighter will also don their hood and helmet. The firefighter will then pick up a 150-foot 1 3/4-inch attack hose bundle and carry it to the third story of the training tower. Upon reaching the third story, the firefighter will drop the hose bundle to the ground. The firefighter will then descend the same stairs, exit the training tower, and walk 10 feet to the final station.

Station 7: Hose Advance and Hose Pull

The firefighter will advance 25 feet with a charged 1 3/4-inch attack line from a kneeling or crawling (i.e. low-profile) position. The firefighter will then pull the same attack line 50 feet from a kneeling stationary position.

During this assessment, the firefighter is in their full PPE (turnout coat and pants, boots, helmet, gloves, and wearing an SCBA on their back). For stations 6 and 7, the firefighter dons their face mask and breathes from the SCBA cylinder.

Firefighters of all ages are allotted a maximum of 12 minutes to complete this PAA.

FIVE CONSIDERATIONS FOR CONDUCTING A PAA

1. Personnel Required to Take the PAA

Only those firefighters qualified by their departments to take an active role in firefighting operations should take the PAA. This includes the following frontline staff: firefighters, driver and operators, and company officers. Chief officers' firefighting roles vary for each fire department, so it should be left up to fire department discretion as to whether or not their chief officers participate.

2. Location of the Assessment

The PAA should be completed outdoors where there is ample space and minimal height restrictions. A training facility or "burn tower" that can accommodate the fireground tasks listed above is an ideal choice. If your department does not have access to a training facility, adapt the PAA to best suit your fire department's needs.

3. Frequency of the Assessment

The assessment should be conducted annually or semiannually. Like the fireground, PAAs are manpower-intensive. For most fire departments, it will not be feasible to conduct a PAA more than once a year.

4. Safety Conditions

Even under optimal safety and weather conditions, injuries and accidents can still happen during a PAA. Firefighters are human. They can trip, fall, or pull a muscle. Therefore, PAA administrators should make great efforts to ensure the highest safety conditions are present. Here are some safety tips for the PAA:

> Ground ladders meant for climbing should be raised to the proper angle, butted, and secured. This can be done with webbing, ropes, etc.

> Abrupt changes in elevation or trip hazards should be minimized. If there are any of these present, paint them with brightly colored spray paint. The PAA supervisor should walk each candidate through the entire course prior to their participation to give an overview. The PAA supervisor will also guide the candidate through the assessment during her participation.

> Ambient temperature and wind conditions should be mild and there should be no precipitation (i. e. avoiding slippery surfaces).

> An ambulance with advanced life support capabilities (preferred) should be placed on stand-by at the PAA. A dedicated EMS crew should be present to assess all participants' vital signs before and after the assessment. If the need should arise, this EMS crew can perform rehabilitation operations (e. g. rehydration, cooling, etc.) and provide medical treatment and transport for injuries or medical emergencies.

5. Manpower Requirement

Conducting a PAA is manpower-intensive. Consider having the following staff present during the assessment:

> **PAA Supervisor** delivers instructions to the candidates, offers guidance during the assessment, and records candidates' times.

> **The EMS Unit** consists of two emergency medical technicians who can assess vital signs and provide rehab support, medical care and transport (if needed).

> **Support Staff** (3 to 5 individuals) assists with resetting the stations, reloading and resetting hose, re-bedding ground ladders, carrying hose bundles, etc.

Remediation

You may be thinking: *"What happens if a firefighter does not finish or pass the PAA?"* If a firefighter does not complete the PAA or does not finish it within the fire department's specified time limit, there are various avenues for remediation. Consider the following set of steps as a possible course of action:

> If a firefighter does not pass the PAA on their **first attempt**, they will have 30 days (but not more than 45) to until they can retest. The candidate is encouraged to focus on improving their fitness through functional exercise and proper nutrition. The candidate should be encouraged to seek fitness guidance and training from a certified personal trainer. The candidate will be mandated to exercise one hour while on duty.

> The candidate will be placed on a "light-duty" assignment, which prohibits them from engaging in active firefighting duties on scene. If the firefighter is an EMT and the fire department provides ambulance services, the firefighter can be temporarily reassigned to the ambulance until they can pass the PAA.

> If the firefighter does not pass the **second attempt**, they will meet with the fire department physician and certified personal trainer to formulate a specific exercise and nutrition "prescription." *All efforts should be made by the fire department's management, labor representatives, and the firefighter to encourage and achieve success.* The candidate will retake the PAA in 90 days (but no longer than 105 days).

> ‣ If the firefighter fails on their **third attempt**, they will be placed on worker's compensation or short term disability. The candidate's continued employment will be decided by representatives of management and labor.

WHAT DOES THE NATIONAL FIRE PROTECTION ASSOCIATION (NFPA) HAVE TO SAY ABOUT FIREFIGHTER FITNESS ASSESSMENTS?

NFPA 1583: Standard on Health-Related Programs for Fire Department Members outlines the following fitness assessment:

1. All members shall participate in a fitness assessment, which is supervised by the fire department health and fitness coordinator.
2. The fitness assessment shall be conducted at least annually.
3. On an annual basis the fire department physician must medically clear all members, as directed by NFPA 1582. After being cleared, these members may participate in the fitness assessment.
4. A pre-assessment questionnaire shall be completed to identify any contraindications for participation (i.e. recent injuries or medical conditions that prohibit participation).
5. Components of an assessment shall include aerobic capacity, body composition, muscular strength, muscular endurance, and flexibility.

WHAT ARE SOME OF THE ORGANIZATIONAL BARRIERS?

As with all things in the fire service that involve change, instituting PAAs at fire departments is bound to draw criticism and resistance. There are different reasons why both management and firefighters could be hesitant about implementing a PAA. Here are some prospective objections and their respective rebuttals:

> **Management may believe that a PAA is costly and "not in the budget."** If the fire department has regular access to a training tower or facility, costs for hosting it should be minimal. PAAs should use the same firefighting equipment that is used on the fireground (e.g. fire hose, ground ladders, PPE, tools, etc.). The need to purchase brand new equipment specifically for the assessment should be nonexistent or minimal. Additionally, previously purchased training props like a rescue mannequin or forcible entry simulator can be repurposed for the PAA.

> **For volunteer departments, a PAA may reduce the number of firefighters who are able to serve in their organization.** Reduced volunteerism is a legitimate concern in today's fire service. However, as we all know, the fireground's physical demands do not discriminate between career and volunteer status, male or female, young or old. Therefore, *all* firefighters must make their fitness a priority, regardless of their monetary compensation. Here is a question for all fire chiefs to consider: *Would you rather find out your firefighters cannot adequately perform during the PAA or while they are at a working fire?* By far, all would chose the former over the latter.

> **Management may view a PAA as a liability** (i.e. one of their firefighters could get injured or become ill during the assessment). We will not beat around the bush: Injuries or acute health events can happen during a PAA. As with any rigorous physical activity related to firefighting, the risk of injury and illness is always present.

> **Firefighters may believe that if they do not pass the PAA they will face discipline, remediation, ridicule, or termination.** It is not the PAA's purpose or goal to "fail" any members or to be used as grounds for termination. Again, it is simply a measurement tool for a firefighter to demonstrate a satisfactory physical fitness level. The PAA should not be something that is extremely easy to pass, nor should it be overly difficult. When all is said and done, it must realistically reflect the physical demands of the fireground.

When a firefighter's personal motivation for fitness and health is lacking, an annual PAA provides them with a form of accountability throughout the year. More importantly, departments must provide functional fitness and nutrition education, provide suitable exercise areas and equipment, and encourage their firefighters to participate in daily exercise.

Just as fire department leadership must establish and communicate job expectations for its members, management must also establish physical fitness expectations for their firefighters. The PAA should be used as a fire department's performance standard all frontline firefighters must achieve.

ACTION STEPS:

1. Learn the core components of a NFPA 1583-compliant PAA. Go to FirefighterFunctionalFitness.com/NFPA1583

2. Research other fire departments for examples of established PAAs and their supporting administrative policies.

3. Form a workgroup to design a basic PAA for your department, and implement it on a voluntary trial basis. Make it fun, and try to get every member of the department from the chief down to the rookie firefighter to participate.

4. Once the final version of the PAA is established, work towards implementing it as a mandatory feature of your department's health and wellness program.

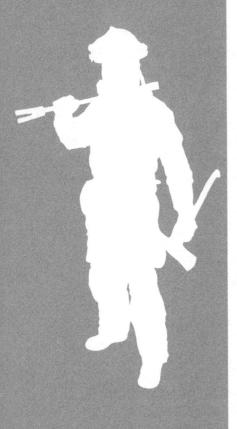

Firefighter Functional Fitness is a practical and comprehensive approach to firefighter fitness that uses real-life activities, positions, and exercises to best prepare firefighters for optimal fireground performance.

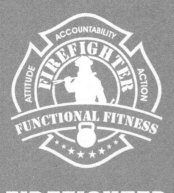

FIREFIGHTER
TOOLBOX

CHAPTER 22

25 FREQUENTLY ASKED QUESTIONS

1. What Is Firefighter Functional Fitness?

Firefighter Functional Fitness is a practical and comprehensive approach to firefighter fitness that uses real-life activities, positions, and exercises to best prepare firefighters for optimal fireground performance. In addition to physical exercise, it also incorporates recovery, hydration, nutrition and a lifestyle of moderation for a holistic approach to fitness—which not only improves fireground performance, but better health overall.

2. Why Is Firefighter Functional Fitness the Best Choice for Optimizing my Fitness as a Firefighter?

A firefighter's physical training must directly reflect the physical intensity of the demanding fireground. While other fitness programs focus on limited aspects of fitness (building muscle mass or strength, weight loss, etc.), *Firefighter Functional Fitness* uses a practical, balanced, and holistic approach to improving a firefighter's fireground performance. Furthermore, **The 4 Pillars** and **The Big 8** of *Firefighter Functional Fitness* provide firefighters with healthy lifestyle principles to promote a long, healthy career *and* retirement.

Just as specialized athletes (gymnasts, football players, basketball players, etc.) tailor their training to meet their specific performance objectives, *Firefighter Functional Fitness* gives firefighters the knowledge and tools to "train like they fight."

3. What Are the 4 Pillars of Firefighter Functional Fitness?

1. Physical fitness
2. Recovery and rest
3. Hydration
4. Nutrition and lifestyle

4. What Are The Big 8 of Firefighter Functional Fitness?

1. Core strength
2. Cardiovascular capacity
3. Flexibility
4. The Push
5. The Pull
6. The Lift
7. The Carry
8. The Drag

5. How Much Should I Exercise Every Week?

Functionally fit firefighters make it a goal to perform at least 150 minutes of vigorous-intensity exercise each week. Vigorous-intensity exercise includes (but is not limited to) functional strength training, flexibility training, core strength exercises, high-intensity interval training and endurance-based cardiovascular training, etc.

6. How Does Firefighter Functional Fitness Combat the Negative Physiological Effects of Firefighting?

Firefighting causes the following physiological effects within the body[38]:

> Muscular and metabolic fatigue
> Dehydration
> Environmental and heat stress
> Cardiovascular strain (increased heart rate, blood pressure, and blood clotting)

Using the principles found in *Firefighter Functional Fitness* directly counteracts these physiological responses by producing the following results:

> Increases muscular strength and endurance
> Decreases level of fatigue and rate to fatigue
> Increases blood plasma volume (i.e. resistance to dehydration)
> Improves thermoregulation and elevated core temperature tolerance
> Increases cardiovascular capacity
> Decreases risk of blood clot formation

7. What Should be the Essential Components of My Weekly Workout Routine?

Core Training

> 2 to 4 times per week
> 10 to 30 minutes per session
> To be combined with another modality (e.g. flexibility, cardio, strength)

Cardiovascular Capacity Training

> 3 or more times per week
> One HIIT session, one EBCT session, and one firefighter circuit training session
> 20 to 60 minutes per session, depending on current conditioning level and intensity of activity

Flexibility Training

> *Dynamic stretching* during warm-ups
> *Static stretching* during cool-downs
> One or more *long flexibility* training sessions per week (e.g. 30 minutes of functional yoga)

Functional Strength Training

> 3 or more times per week (one upper-body session, one lower-body session, one total-body session)
> 20 to 32 total sets per session (e.g. upper-body push and pull session: 10 to 16 sets of pushing exercises, 10 to 16 sets of pulling exercises)
> Upper-body sessions combining pushing, pulling, and carrying exercises are ideal
> Lower-body sessions combining lifting, carrying, and

dragging exercises are ideal

> Total-body sessions combining all elements of The Big 8 to work the upper and lower body, as well as the core.

8. Does Firefighting at the Fireground Count as Exercise?

Yes! Whether you spend your time "making the stretch" on the fireground or you are "making yourself stretch" in the gym, you are engaging in exercise. As long as you are *doing work* on the fireground (pulling or advancing hose lines, carrying heavy equipment, forcible entry, search and rescue, etc.), you are simultaneously elevating your heart rate and breathing rate, as well as providing resistance to your muscles.

9. Which Modalities Are Best for Functional Strength Training?

> **Firefighting equipment**: SCBA harness and cylinder, fire hose, hand tools, hydraulic tools, saws, rope, ladders, etc.

> **Free weights**: Dumbbells, barbells, and kettlebells

> **Bodyweight exercises**: Push-ups, pull-ups, core exercises, air squats, lunges, etc.

> **Cable machines**

> **Resistance bands**

> **Medicine balls**

> **Suspension strap systems**: TRX® or WOSS® straps

Functionally fit firefighters also focus on executing compound movements. These are movements that improve balance, coordination, and incorporate a total-body workout. Squats, deadlifts, and kettlebell push-press are examples of compound movements.

10. Are Traditional Weight Machines Effective in Improving Functional Fitness?

Stationary weight machines (bench press, "pec-deck," leg curl, leg extension, etc.) will increase your muscular strength, but these are the least-preferred method of improving your functional strength. These machines typically yield unnatural, nonfunctional movements for firefighters. Furthermore, they emphasize isolation movements (bicep curl, tricep extension) over compound movements. When possible, choose to use exercises that incorporate the core: push-ups, standing cable chest press, standing overhead press, inverted rows, standing/kneeling cable rows, kettlebell swings, etc.

11. Should I Work out While On-Duty at the Firehouse?

The short and simple answer: *YES*.

However, there are numerous variables that firefighters must consider, including:

> - High call volume may interrupt workout sessions
> - Physical intensity of hands-on training during the same shift
> - Firefighters could respond to a working fire at any time

While we encourage every firefighter to exercise at the firehouse, we also recommend that they be smart in their approach. Remember, activities such as company training and performing tasks like lifting patients and carrying equipment count as exercise, too. If any of the variables above are a concern, firefighters may want to consider lighter-intensity workouts at the firehouse: quick sets of bodyweight exercises "on the hour" (ex: 10 push-ups and 10 air squats every hour for 8 to 10 hours), endurance-based cardiovascular training, functional yoga, foam rolling, etc.

12. Should I Exercise While Wearing my Firefighting Protective Ensemble?

Perhaps the central-most concept of *Firefighter Functional Fitness* is to "practice like you play" and "train like you fight."

Functionally fit firefighters *occasionally* wear their turnout gear, helmet, gloves, SCBA, and mask during exercise sessions to replicate the realism of a physically demanding fireground. They know that their protective ensemble restricts movement and range of motion, increases heart rate and energy expenditure, and also develops muscle memory and skill proficiency.

If you are just starting out in your *Firefighter Functional Fitness* journey, we recommend that you ease into working out while wearing your firefighter protective ensemble. Please read Chapter 16 *Workout Programming: Putting it All Together* to know how to progress through different stages of exercising in your protective ensemble.

As a rule of thumb, functionally fit firefighters will make it a goal to complete one firefighter training circuit per week while wearing their protective ensemble.

13. What Is the Best Kind of Cardiorespiratory Exercise for Firefighters to Do?

Functionally fit firefighters combine high-intensity interval training and strength training into firefighter training circuits. The ideal firefighter circuit typically consists of a firefighter wearing their protective ensemble and completing 4 to 6 fireground-related stations into a circuit.

Here is an example of a firefighter circuit:

1. Strike a tire with a sledgehammer for 30 seconds
2. Drag a rescue mannequin or a tire for 50 feet
3. Carry a ground ladder 50 feet, then raise it against a building
4. Crawl 50 feet
5. Drag large diameter supply hose 100 feet (with coupling over the shoulder)
6. Ascend and descend stairs for one minute

Depending on your current level of conditioning, repeat the circuit for a total of 3 to 6 rounds, either wearing gym clothes or with your firefighting protective ensemble.

14. When and How Should I Stretch: Before or After a Workout?

Dynamic stretching during warm-ups, before a workout. Dynamic stretches use repetitive motion to elongate and warm up muscles. Examples include the dowel rod chest openers, arm circles, lunges, air squats, etc.

Static stretching during cool-downs, after a workout. These are the "reach and hold" stretches that are held for at least 30 seconds.

Examples include the seated "sit and reach" hamstring stretch, butterfly groin stretch, etc.

Longer flexibility training sessions (e.g. 30 to 60 minutes of functional yoga) should be used at least once per week. If yoga is chosen as the medium, just make sure it is basic it its movements. There is no need to contort yourself into pretzel-like positions.

15. How Do I Increase my Flexibility?

Functionally fit firefighters use three primary methods of increasing their flexibility:

1. **Cardiovascular capacity training**: Most back pain, aches and muscle stiffness result from being overly sedentary. Regular *movement* is key to improving flexibility because it increases muscular elasticity and joint range of motion.

2. **Regular Stretching**: Using dynamic stretching before workouts and static stretching during cool downs has been proven to improve flexibility. If muscles are overly tight, use self-myofascial release (foam rolling) as an adjunct to loosen them up.

> "An object at rest will remain at rest unless acted on by an unbalanced force. An object in motion continues in motion with the same speed and in the same direction unless acted upon by an unbalanced force."
> —Isaac Newton

3. **Functional Yoga**: A stand-alone flexibility training session with functional yoga incorporates aspects of stretching, balance, core strength, muscular strength, cardiovascular capacity training, and more.

16. If I Am Short on Time, What Kind of Workout Will Give me the Most Bang for my Buck?

To maximally impact cardiovascular capacity and simultaneously improve muscular strength, functionally fit firefighters combine *high-intensity interval training* and *functional strength training*. If you are short on time, complete a strength training circuit with bodyweight exercises that uses HIIT.

HIIT and functional strength training circuit:

1. Push-ups
2. Walking lunges
3. Pull-ups
4. Air squats
5. Crawling
6. Squat jumps
7. Hanging leg raises
8. Side lunges

At each station, do as many repetitions as you can during the high-intensity periods (30 seconds in duration). Use the 30-second recovery periods. Repeat the circuit for a total of 15 to 30 minutes.

17. What Is a Simple, Low-impact Exercise That Every Firefighter Should Do?

Crawling is an incredibly beneficial Firefighter Functional Fitness movement for the following reasons:

> It simultaneously builds cardiovascular capacity and total-body strength (upper, lower, and core).

> It is low impact.

> It requires no equipment and can be done anywhere.

> It can be combined with other exercises to optimize workout effectiveness (e.g. crawl 50 feet then sprint, drag, push, pull, or carry back to the start).

18. What Are Basic Principles for Losing Weight?

For firefighters who want to get their weight under control, put these principles into action:

1. **Focus on eating the right foods** (foods with healthy fats, carbohydrates, proteins, and fiber), instead of placing unrealistic restrictions on your daily nutrition.

2. *All calories are not created equal.* There is a big difference between 200 calories from a serving of almonds and 200 calories from a soda. The former has healthy fiber, protein, carbohydrates, and fat; the latter is nothing but sugar and empty calories (which will immediately be

converted to fat once they reach the liver).

3. ***Start small***. Making small, incremental changes yields greater long-term success because they are easier to adopt and stick with.

4. **Instead of "starving yourself" or eating 2 to 3 very large meals, eat 3 medium-sized meals with 2 to 3 medium-sized snacks throughout the day.** Only eating 2 to 3 large meals alone leads to a rollercoaster response of spiking blood sugars and massive insulin release, which is counterproductive to weight loss.

5. **For the first 1 to 2 weeks, measure all of the food you eat and record it in a food diary.** Being more aware of the foods we eat helps us to make better choices.

6. **Drink plenty of water to stay hydrated (at least 13 cups for men, 9 cups for women).**

7. **Cut or reduce "empty," non-beneficial calories from your diet: sugar, soda, alcohol, and refined carbohydrates.**

8. ***Natural foods* should always be the first choice over highly-processed, preservative-laden foods.** The latter have been proven to have higher amounts of calories and do not promote satiety.

9. **High-intensity interval training burns more calories and fat than long-duration, low-intensity exercise.** HIIT also results in greater "excess post-oxygen consumption" after exercise and therefore boosts the body's metabolism levels—*burning more calories*.

10. **Don't eat directly out of the container!** Whether it is a bag of potato chips, box of crackers, or a carton of ice cream, choose a modest portion and put it in a bowl. Then seal up the bag or container and put it out of sight. When we eat directly out of the container, we lose track of our portion sizes, leading us to overeat and consume excessive calories.

18. Which Foods Help Me Stay Fuller, Longer?

Foods that promote satiety include fiber-rich foods, healthy fats, and lean proteins.

1. Fiber-Rich Foods

> **Fresh fruit**: Pears, apples, raspberries, bananas, blueberries, oranges, and strawberries

> **Dried fruit**: Prunes, dried figs, raisins, and dried apricots

> **Vegetables**: Artichoke hearts, pea varieties, leafy greens (spinach, mustard, collard), corn, broccoli, brussels sprouts, onions, and sweet potatoes

> **Legumes**: Chickpeas, pea varieties, lentils, beans, and soybeans

> **Whole grains**: Oatmeal (steel-cut or old-fashioned, not instant), oat bran, popcorn, whole wheat, farro, millet, quinoa, brown rice (not white), rye, spelt, and wild rice

> **Nuts and seeds**: Flaxseed, chia seeds, almonds, pistachios, pumpkin seeds, and sesame seeds

2. Healthy Fats

> **Monounsaturated fat**: Avocados, nuts, oils: olive, peanut, and sesame

> **Polyunsaturated fat**: Walnuts, leafy vegetables, soy, tofu, salmon, trout, and mackerel

> **Saturated fat**: Natural animal proteins, eggs, butter, and coconut oil

3. Proteins

> **Poultry**: Grilled or baked, not breaded and fried

> **Fish**: Salmon, trout, and herring (preferably wild caught, not farm-raised)

> **Beef, pork, and lamb**

> **Game meats**: Venison, buffalo, elk, etc.

> **Nuts**: Almonds, peanuts, walnuts, and cashews *(raw or lightly salted, and non-roasted, if possible)*

> **Legumes**: Beans, lentils, chickpeas, soybeans, and tofu

> **Low-fat Greek yogurt**

19. What Are Some Healthy Choices for Snacks Throughout the Day?

> - Nuts: Almonds, peanuts, walnuts, pecans, pistachios, flaxseed, sesame seeds, etc.
> - Natural nut butters: Peanut, almond, etc.
> - Fruit (high in fiber and with low glycemic index): Pears, apples, cherries, bananas, peach, and citrus fruits (e.g. oranges, grapefruit)
> - Salsa or guacamole with corn tortilla chips
> - Granola with whole grains (low in sugar)
> - Greek yogurt
> - Veggies with hummus
> - Low-sodium meat jerky (e.g. beef, turkey, chicken, etc.)

20. Are Carbohydrates Bad for Me? How Many Carbohydrates Should I Eat Every day?

Contrary to the popular *no-carb* and *low-carb* diet fads, not all carbohydrates are bad for you. Just like luxury sports cars need the highest-quality performance fuel, functionally fit firefighters need high-quality carbohydrates to fuel their performance. *Quality* carbohydrates provide glucose to the body, which is then converted into energy.

The best kinds of carbohydrates are fruits and vegetables with plenty of fiber, whole grains, and those with a low to moderate glycemic index.

If you have been diagnosed with diabetes or insulin resistance, consult with your physician and a registered dietitian to formulate a customized nutritional plan for carbohydrate consumption.

21. How Much Protein Should I Eat Every day? Is Too Much Protein Bad for Me?

For daily protein intake, the National Academy of Sports Medicine recommends 0.5-0.8 grams/pound for *strength athletes*[39]. A functionally fit firefighter's level of performance most closely resembles that of a *strength athlete*. For a 200-pound firefighter who takes their fitness seriously and works out 5 to 6 days per week, this translates to 100 to 160 grams of quality protein per day.

Most bodybuilders will tell you that *"You can never eat enough protein."* It is true that protein is one of the building blocks of adding muscle mass, but an increase in calories and carbohydrates is equally, if not *more* important. However, we must remember that the primary goal of *Firefighter Functional Fitness* is to optimize performance, not to solely focus on muscle mass and body composition.

Excessive protein intake (especially from the wrong sources) is harmful to our bodies. Too much protein can cause kidney disease, weight gain, body fat gain, dehydration, cancer, and shortened life expectancy.

22. How Does Dehydration Affect Firefighters?

Simply put, dehydration increases cardiovascular strain. When combined with a firefighter's extreme physical workload and hot environment, the risk of a sudden cardiac event or death increases by more than 100 times during firefighting activities. Here are some specific effects on the body.

Dehydration's *physiological* effects:

> Blood plasma volume decreases
> Blood viscosity (thickness) increases
> Skin blood flow decreases
> Sweating decreases
> Decrease in body heat release and subsequent dissipation
> Core temperature increases
> Muscle glycogen use increases (depleting muscle energy and capacity)

Dehydration's effects on *physical performance*:

> VO_2 max (cardiovascular capacity) decreases by 5 percent for a fluid loss of 3 percent body mass. For warm environments (e.g. the fireground), VO_2 max decreases even more. Even for normally-hydrated firefighters, environmental

heat stress can reduce VO_2 max by 7 percent.

> The amount of time to exhaustion is reduced by 45 percent for 2.5 percent body weight dehydration. Therefore, dehydration reduces the length of time we can effectively perform on the fireground.

Cardiovascular effects of dehydration:

> Decrease in blood plasma volume

> Decrease in cardiac output (the amount of blood pumped by the heart every minute)

> Increase in the heart's oxygen demand and metabolic workload because it has to beat faster and more forcefully

> Increase in blood's viscosity (thickness)

> Increase in the formation of blood clots and blockages

23. How Much Water Should I Drink Every Day?

The National Academy of Sports Medicine recommends drinking the following amounts of water each day:

> 3 liters (approximately 13 cups) for men

> 2.2 liters (approximately 9 cups) for women

These figures are for average-sized, sedentary men and women who do not operate in extreme environments.

Since functionally fit firefighters are performance athletes who regularly experience heat stress and elevated core temperatures, they should aim to exceed these baseline recommendations. Depending on the number of physically demanding alarms a firefighter responds to, their daily fluid intake may far surpass the amounts above.

24. What Are 3 Ways to Reduce and Prevent Back Pain?

Contrary to popular belief, the majority of back pain isn't caused by "doing too much," it is actually a result of *not doing enough*. A sedentary lifestyle (i.e. excessive sitting) is the primary culprit for back pain.

There are 3 primary ways to reduce and prevent back pain: *frequent exercise, building core strength,* and *regular flexibility training.* Each of these elements plays their part in increasing muscular flexibility and joint range of motion, as well as keeping our weight under control.

25. What Are the Most Important National Fire Protection Association Standards for Firefighter Fitness and Health?

NFPA 1500–Standard on Fire Department Occupational Safety and Health Program

NFPA 1582–Standard on Occupational Medical Programs for Fire Departments

NFPA 1583–Standard on Health-Related Fitness Programs for Fire Department Members

NFPA 1584–Standard on Rehabilitation Process for Members During Emergency Operations and Training Exercises

REFERENCES

1. International Association of Firefighters. (2013). Heart Disease in the Fire Service. Retrieved from https://www.iaff.org/hs/PDF/HeartDiseaseManual_2013.pdf

2. Clark, M. A., Lucett, S. C., & Sutton, B. G. (Eds). (2014). *NASM Essentials of Personal Fitness Training* (4th ed.). Burlington, MA: Jones & Bartlett Learning

3. Peate, W. F., Bates, G., Lunda, K., Francis, S., & Bellamy, K. (2007). Core strength: A new model for injury prediction and prevention. *Journal of Occupational Medicine and Toxicology*, 2(3). Retrieved from http://www.ncbi.nlm.nih.gov/pmc/articles/PMC1865378/

4. Gergley, J.C. (2013). Acute effect of passive static stretching on lower-body strength in moderately trained men [Abstract]. *Journal of Strength and Conditioning Research*, 27(4). Retrieved from http://www.ncbi.nlm.nih.gov/pubmed/22692125

5. Mayo Clinic. (2015). Yoga: Fight stress and find serenity. Retrieved from http://www.mayoclinic.org/healthy-lifestyle/stress-management/in-depth/yoga/art-20044733

6. International Association of Firefighters. (2015). Back Injuries and the Firefighter. Retrieved from http://www.iaff.org/hs/resi/backpain.asp

7. Lindberg, A. (2014). Firefighters' physical work capacity. Retrieved from http://umu.diva-portal.org/smash/get/diva2:719114/FULLTEXT01.pdf

8. Perroni, F., Guidetti, L., and Cignitti, L. (2014). Psychophysiological Responses of Firefighters to Emergencies: A Review. *The Open Sports Sciences Journal*, 7(1). Retrieved from http://www.researchgate.net/publication/264375959_Psychophysiological_Responses_of_Firefighters_to_Emergencies_A_Review

9. Eves, N. D., Jones, R. L., & Peterson, S. R. (2005). The Influence of the Self-Contained Breathing Apparatus (SCBA) on Ventilatory Function and Maximal Exercise. Retrieved from http://journals.humankinetics.com/AcuCustom/Sitename/Documents/DocumentItem/5045.pdf

10. National Heart, Lung, and Blood Institute. (2012) Why Is Sleep Important? Retrieved from http://www.nhlbi.nih.gov/health/health-topics/topics/sdd/why

11. Shin, M.S. & Sung Y.H. (2014). Effects on Massage on Muscular Strength and Proprioception after Exercise-Induced Muscle Damage. *Journal of Strength and Conditioning Research* 29(8), 2255-60.

12. Horn, G.P., DeBlois, J., Shalmyeva, I., & Smith. D.L. (2012). Quantifying dehydration in the Fire Service using field measures and novel devices. Pre-hospital Emergency Care, 16(3): 347-355

13. Jeukendrup, A. & Gleeson, M. (2009). *Sports Nutrition: An Introduction to Energy Production and Performance* (2nd ed.), Champaign, IL: Human Kinetics

14. International Association of Firefighters. (2013). Heart Disease in the Fire Service. Retrieved from https://www.iaff.org/hs/PDF/HeartDiseaseManual_2013.pdf

15. Batmanghelidj, F. (2005). *Obesity Cancer & Depression: Their Common Cause & Natural Cure*. Falls Church, VA: Global Health Solutions

16. National Institutes of Health. (2016). "Facts about polyunsaturated fats." Retrieved from https://www.nlm.nih.gov/medlineplus/ency/patientinstructions/000747.htm

17. Mercola, J. (2009). 7 Reasons to Eat More Saturated Fat. Retrieved from http://articles.mercola.com/sites/articles/archive/2009/09/22/7-reasons-to-eat-more-saturated-fat.aspx

18. Mayo Clinic. (2014). Trans fat is double trouble for your heart health. Retrieved from http://www.mayoclinic.org/trans-fat/art-20046114

[19.] Harvard School of Health. (2015). Carbohydrates.
Retrieved from http://www.hsph.harvard.edu/nutritionsource/carbohydrates/

[20.] Clark, M. A., Lucett, S. C., & Sutton, B. G. (Eds). (2014). *NASM Essentials of Personal Fitness Training* (4th ed.). Burlington, MA: Jones & Bartlett Learning

[21.] Mayo Clinic. (2013). Healthy diet: Do you follow dietary guidelines?
Retrieved from http://www.mayoclinic.org/healthy-lifestyle/nutrition-and-healthy-eating/in-depth/how-to-eat-healthy/art-20046590

[22.] National Institutes of Health. (2016). Fiber.
Retrieved from https://www.nlm.nih.gov/medlineplus/ency/article/002470.htm

[23.] American Institute for Cancer Research. (n.d). AICR's Foods that Fight Cancer.
Retrieved from http://www.aicr.org/foods-that-fight-cancer/

[24.] Rhoades, J., & Favorite, K.C. (2014). A Fire Department Guide to Implementing NFPA 1582. Retrieved from https://www.iafc.org/files/1SAFEhealthSHS/shs_FDguideToImplementingNPFA1582.pdf

[25.] National Fire Protection Association. (2007). *NFPA 1582: Standard on comprehensive medical program for fire departments.* Quincy, MA: National Fire Protection Association

[26.] United States Fire Administration. (2014). Firefighter Fatalities in the United States in 2014. Retrieved from: https://www.usfa.fema.gov/downloads/pdf/publications/ff_fat14.pdf

[27.] International Association of Firefighters. (2013). Heart Disease in the Fire Service.
Retrieved from https://www.iaff.org/hs/PDF/HeartDiseaseManual_2013.pdf

[28.] Ibid.

[29.] Ibid.

[30.] Ibid.

[31.] Ibid.

[32.] Ibid.

[33.] Ibid.

[34.] Centers for Disease Control and Prevention. (2015). Quitting Smoking. Retrieved from http://www.cdc.gov/tobacco/data_statistics/fact_sheets/cessation/quitting/

[35.] Clark, S. (2007). Firefighter Safety During Overhaul at the Manhattan Fire Department. Retrieved from http://nfa.usfa.fema.gov/pdf/efop/efo40819.pdf

[36.] International Association of Firefighters. (2013). Heart Disease in the Fire Service.
Retrieved from https://www.iaff.org/hs/PDF/HeartDiseaseManual_2013.pdf

[37.] Smith, D., Liebig, J.P., Steward, N.M, & Fehling, P.C.. (2010). Sudden Cardiac Events in the Fire Service: Understanding the Cause and Mitigating the Risks.
Retrieved from https://www.skidmore.edu/responder/documents/DHS-Sudden-Cardiac-Events-Report.pdf.

[38.] Smith, D., Liebig, J.P., Steward, N.M, & Fehling, P.C. (2010). Sudden Cardiac Events in the Fire Service: Understanding the Cause and Mitigating the Risks.
Retrieved from https://www.skidmore.edu/responder/documents/DHS-Sudden-Cardiac-Events-Report.pdf.

[39.] Clark, M. A., Lucett, S. C., & Sutton, B. G. (Eds). (2014). *NASM Essentials of Personal Fitness Training* (4th ed.). Burlington, MA: Jones & Bartlett Learning

APPENDIX A. FITNESS, NUTRITION, HEALTH, AND WELLNESS RESOURCES

This section is dedicated to resources that can help in your *Firefighter Functional Fitness* journey. Please visit these websites for valuable information on firefighter fitness, nutrition, health, and wellness.

Firefighter Functional Fitness: FirefighterFunctionalFitness.com

BlastMask: BlastMask.com

Everyone Goes Home: EveryoneGoesHome.com

Firefighter Behavioral Health Alliance: ffbha.org

Firefighter Cancer Support Network: FirefighterCancerSupport.org

Firefighter Dynamic Performance Training: FD-PT.com

Firefighter Toolbox: FirefighterToolbox.com

Fit for Duty Consulting: FitForDutyConsulting.com

Harvard School of Public Health: hsph.harvard.edu/nutritionsource/healthy-eating-plate/

Illinois Fire Service Institute: fsi.illinois.edu

International Association of Fire Chiefs: iafc.org

International Association of Firefighters: iaff.org

International Firefighter Cancer Foundation: ffcancer.org

Mayo Clinic: MayoClinic.org

National Academy of Sports Medicine: nasm.org

National Fallen Firefighters Foundation: FireHero.org

National Institute for Occupational Safety and Health (NIOSH): cdc.gov/niosh/fire/

National Strength and Conditioning Association: ncsa.com

National Volunteer Fire Council: nvfc.org

National Volunteer Fire Council Heart Healthy Firefighter Program: http://www.nvfc.org/programs/heart-healthy-firefighter-program

Nutrition.gov: nutrition.gov

Safe Call Now: safecallnow.org

Share the Load Program: nvfc.org/programs/share-the-load-program/

The First Twenty: TheFirstTwenty.org

United States Fire Administration: usfa.fema.gov

FIREFIGHTER
T O O L B O X

FIREFIGHTERTOOLBOX.COM

Firefighter Toolbox is an online training resource and community for firefighters and officers who want to take their skills to the next level. The purpose of Firefighter Toolbox is to build better firefighters and leaders to positively impact the future of the fire service. Firefighter Toolbox provides high-quality books, online training materials, videos, audio programs, and more for firefighters and officers to learn from and to share with their crews.

MUST READ SPECIAL REPORT BY FIREFIGHTER TOOLBOX

THE BIG 5: The 5 Biggest Mistakes Firefighters Make and How to Avoid Them. This special report outlines the five biggest mistakes firefighters make and how to avoid them.

Learn more at FirefighterToolbox.com/Big5

FIREFIGHTER PREPLAN BOOK OR AUDIO PROGRAM

Firefighter Preplan **is the ultimate guidebook for thriving as a firefighter**. In this program, you will discover the secrets of great firefighters that have never been shared in a book before. You will be given the strategies and tactics of great and respected firefighters and a plan for how you implement it.

Specifics you will learn:

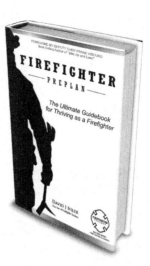

- 17 strategies of great and respected firefighters
- 10 tactics used by great and respected firefighters
- How to build a respected reputation among firefighters
- The 4 respect-killers for firefighters
- The top 3 most-hated firefighter behaviors
- The 3 destructive C's in the fire service
- The Firefighter Motto of successful firefighters
- How to be like the fire
- Firefighter Preplan implementation steps
- The Firefighter Training Success Diamond
- Action steps for each strategy and tactic
- How to deal with the career and life storms of a fire service career
- And much more!

Firefighter Preplan provides the opportunity to learn what the best of the best in our business do. *Firefighter Preplan* eliminates the constraints of previous up-and-coming firefighters.

Regardless of where you live, where you are stationed, what your gender or nationality is, you can have access to the wisdom of great firefighters with *Firefighter Preplan.* Learn the attitudes, mindsets, behaviors, strategies and tactics of great firefighters in *Firefighter Preplan* to take your firefighting career and skills to the next level and to reach your God-given potential.

Learn more at FirefighterPreplan.com

FIREFIGHTER TOOLBOX PODCAST

Listen to the interviews and training that Firefighter Toolbox and David J. Soler provide on the podcast.

Learn more at FirefighterToolbox.com/about

FIREFIGHTER TOOLBOX 5-MINUTE CLINICS

One-page PDF training documents for study and company trainings.

Learn more at FirefighterToolbox.com/5minuteclinic

ABOUT THE AUTHORS
DAN KERRIGAN

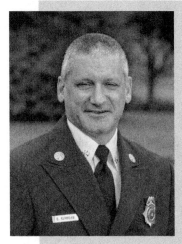

Dan Kerrigan is a 29-year fire service veteran, assistant fire marshal/deputy emergency management coordinator, and Department Health and Fitness coordinator for the East Whiteland Township Department of Codes and Life Safety in Chester County, Pa. Dan also serves as the director of The First Twenty's Firefighter Functional Training Advisory Panel, and he acts as an IAFC-VCOS representative for the National Near Miss Reporting Program.

He is a passionate and knowledgeable advocate for firefighter health and wellness. In addition to presenting nationally at the Fire Department Instructors Conference, the National Volunteer Fire Council (NVFC), and Firehouse World, he is a local Russian kettlebells instructor in his community. Dan has conducted original research on firefighter functional fitness as well as other fire service leadership topics. Dan works closely with the International Association of Fire Chiefs (IAFC), National Fallen Firefighters Foundation (NFFF), and NVFC on strategies to improve fitness and reduce health-related LODDs in the fire service.

Dan is a graduate of the National Fire Academy's Executive Fire Officer Program, a credentialed Chief Fire Officer (CFO), and holds a master's degree in Executive Fire Service Leadership. He is a Pennsylvania State Fire Academy Suppression Level instructor as well as an adjunct professor at Anna Maria College, Neumann University, and Immaculata University. He is a contributor to Fire Engineering Magazine, Firehouse Magazine, Firefighter Toolbox, Hooks and Hooligans, the IAFC, and the NVFC. He was the 2014 recipient of the IAFC-VCOS Emerging Leader Scholarship sponsored by Dr. Richard Gasaway.

Contact Dan at *dankerrigan911@gmail.com*. Connect with him on Facebook and LinkedIn, and follow him on Twitter: @dankerrigan911 and @FirefighterFFit

JIM MOSS

Jim Moss is a career fire officer with the Metro West Fire Protection District of St. Louis County, Missouri. Jim is an active member of the fitness committee at Metro West FPD and he is also a member of *The First Twenty's* Firefighter Functional Training Advisory Panel. He is a certified personal trainer through the National Academy of Sports Medicine. His passion for fitness and health goes beyond his time in the fire service, even dating back to his youth.

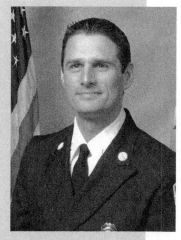

Jim is a regular contributor to FirefighterToolbox.com, and he has contributed to FireEngineering.com, TheFirstTwenty.org, and FireTrainingToolbox.com. He has presented Firefighter Functional Fitness at FDIC, Firehouse World, International Society of Fire Service Instructors (ISFSI), and online through the IAFC/NVFC. Jim is also a member of the ISFSI. He possesses multiple degrees, two of which are in Fire Science from Columbia Southern University.

Contact him at *jimmoss911@gmail.com*. Connect with him on Facebook, LinkedIn, and follow him on Twitter: @jimmoss911and @FirefighterFFit

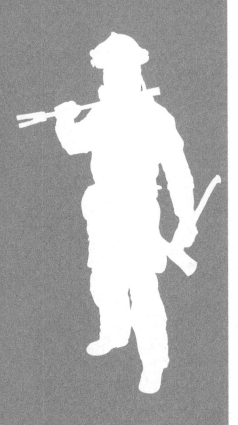

THANK YOU FOR YOUR PURCHASE!

As a bonus to supplement your health and fitness journey, go to FirefighterFunctionalFitness.com/BookBonus to get these valuable resources.

1. Special Report: The 10 Biggest Mistakes Firefighters Make With Their Fitness.

2. An interview with the authors on tips for getting started and staying motivated.

FirefighterFunctionalFitness.com/
BookBonus

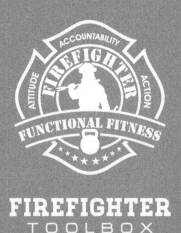

FIREFIGHTER
TOOLBOX

Printed in Great Britain
by Amazon

26671263R00178